The Mind-Body Cure

The Mind-Body Cure

Heal Your Pain, Anxiety, and Fatigue by Controlling Chronic Stress

BAL PAWA, MD

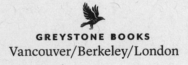

GREYSTONE BOOKS
Vancouver/Berkeley/London

Greystone Books Ltd.
greystonebooks.com

Cataloguing data available from Library and Archives Canada
ISBN 978-1-77164-579-9 (pbk)
ISBN 978-1-77164-580-5 (epub)

Editing by Lucy Kenward
Copy editing by Rowena Rae
Proofreading by Dawn Loewen
Indexing by Stephen Ullstrom
Cover design by Belle Wuthrich
Text design by Fiona Siu
Illustrations by Belle Wuthrich

Printed and bound in Canada on FSC® certified paper at Friesens. The FSC®
label means that materials used for the product have been responsibly sourced.

Greystone Books gratefully acknowledges the Musqueam, Squamish, and
Tsleil-Waututh peoples on whose land our Vancouver head office is located.

Greystone Books thanks the Canada Council for the Arts, the British
Columbia Arts Council, the Province of British Columbia through the Book
Publishing Tax Credit, and the Government of Canada for supporting our
publishing activities.

Canada

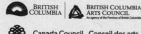
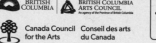

BRITISH
COLUMBIA

BRITISH COLUMBIA
ARTS COUNCIL
An agency of the Province of British Columbia

Canada Council
for the Arts

Conseil des arts
du Canada

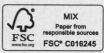

MIX
Paper from
responsible sources
FSC® C016245

Contents

Preface   vii
Introduction   1

1. Mind Your Mind   7
2. Mind Your Brain   36
3. Mind Your Breath   64
4. Mind Your Gut   89
5. Mind Your Movement   121
6. Mind Your Heart   159
7. Mind Your Sleep   188
8. Mind Your Immune System   219
9. The REFRAME Toolkit: 251
    Seven Tools to Re-set Your Health

Acknowledgments   265
Appendix A: Gut Health Assessment   268
Appendix B: Supplements   273
Notes   284
Selected Bibliography   297
Index   308

Preface

GLANCED IN THE rearview mirror just in time to see a large black truck hurtling toward my car at full speed. I automatically braced for the impact, which it turned out I had grossly underestimated. The driver was looking sideways, oblivious to the little car stopped in front of him waiting for another car to turn left.

I was on my way home from the hospital obstetrical ward after an extra-long day delivering a baby whose mom had endured a difficult labor. The birth had ended happily, and I was recalling how that big, beautiful baby boy had cried at the top of his lungs to signal his healthy entry into the world. This is the most satisfying sound for both new mothers and their medical practitioners. Watching the parents bond with their baby and being privileged to be a part of that milestone were rewarding aspects of my career.

I loved managing my role as a busy physician with my other role as the mother of two young, beautiful children and looking forward to another one on the way. As my thoughts turned to the squeals of delight I'd hear from my children when I got home, the loud squeal of tires abruptly interrupted and I heard a sickening crunch. The truck had lunged up over my car, shattering the back window and landing threateningly close to my head before coming to a stop. The impact happened so suddenly and so powerfully that my little white Honda lurched forward, hitting the car in front of me before being pushed into oncoming traffic in the other lane. With screeching tires, scraping metal, and blaring horns all around me, I felt searing pain in my right arm as I grasped at the stick shift to gain some control. My body had become a human missile: I must have hit my head on the side window and my chest on the steering wheel. I could barely breathe. Fortunately, the seat belt restrained me and saved me from going through the windshield.

I struggled to regain focus and understand what had just happened. Many onlookers were staring in horror at my car, now folded like an accordion. My body was wedged in the front seat between the mangled metal pieces in the front and back. I felt nauseous—my head was spinning and I retched from intense pain. I heard sirens in the distance, the all-too-familiar sound of an ambulance, which was being sent to help me. I could not get out of my car and I vaguely recall emergency responders asking me, "Do you know where you are? What is your name? Do you know what day it is? Are you in pain?" A large crowd was gathering, and all traffic on the busy street had come to a standstill. My head was spinning. And then, total blackout!

The next thing I recall, I was being wheeled into the emergency room of the same hospital I had left an hour before as a physician. The neck brace prevented me from turning sideways to see the familiar surroundings. I could only gaze at the ceiling, and I realized that while working as a physician I had never looked up there. Lying on a stretcher as a helpless patient, I had a whole new perspective. The role reversal was scary and sobering.

"Does it hurt to breathe? Do you know where you are? Were you wearing a seat belt?" A young ER doctor fired questions at me while efficiently checking my vitals. Confused and dizzy from the pain, my mind floated back and forth between panic and denial. I knew I was alive: hands were poking and prodding me and placing cold stethoscopes on my chest and abdomen. I felt the sharp jab of a needle as they started an IV in my arm and I made a mental note of all the patients I'd had to poke repeatedly when I was an inexperienced medical student.

Various technicians prepared me for X-rays and fired more questions at me: "When was your last period? Is there a possibility you could be pregnant?" I was pregnant! Fear and panic ran through me about the well-being of my unborn child. I cringed at the thought of radiation penetrating my uterus. The hospital notified my husband who rushed to my side, but it seemed like several hours before I could speak coherently or organize my thoughts to piece together what had just happened. Within a few hours, our lives were turned upside down, and we had to face a brand new future that fate had decided for us.

That night was the start of a dark chapter in my life, but it ultimately shaped who I am today, both personally and professionally. The next seven years brought constant pain, grief, sadness, sleepless nights, and drastic changes to my life as I had known it. The pain from fractured ribs, a dislocated shoulder, torn rotator cuff, multiple soft-tissue injuries, and whiplash penetrated to my core, and over-the-counter medications rarely relieved it. In the ordeal, I lost my baby and I felt terribly sad and depressed for our loss, which only added to the emotional and physical anguish of the accident. On top of that, I would wake up with terrifying nightmares, as my nervous system relived the horrific accident over and over. The unstable shoulder meant I could not lift my two-year-old daughter out of her crib or pick her up when she fell, and I could not play ball with my son; I longed to be a hands-on, fun-loving mom again. I could no longer do what I loved professionally: deliver babies and look after my patients. My wholesome life as I had known it was over. The person I knew was gone.

Over the next few years, I had multiple injections of steroids and anesthetics into my shoulder and trigger points in my neck, none of which offered long-lasting benefits. The scar tissue that built up—after the initial fractures healed—compressed the nerves and blood vessels in my right arm, and my arm became numb and painful with activity. I eventually required more surgery. I woke up the day after my third surgery in severe pain, with a chest tube in place, only to find out that my lung had punctured and collapsed during the delicate operation. Tears rolled down my cheeks as I lay on a hospital bed feeling hopeless and defeated.

What had happened to Superwoman? That was the name my mother had fondly called me when she saw me in action. I was the one who came to the rescue, the one who took care of everyone else. I was the one who fixed things. I had never needed to be rescued or fixed. Everything I had previously taken for granted—my health, my career, my contagious energy—was gone.

My nightstand became my personal pharmacy, filled with painkillers, sleeping pills, anti-inflammatories, muscle relaxants and ointments for pain, ice packs, and heating pads. My children couldn't understand why Mommy couldn't play with them anymore. My husband supported me tremendously, but he had to witness me trying to pick up the pieces of my "super" life as he struggled to look after his patients, care for me, and look after the children. I saw so many specialists over the next few years—including a neurologist, rheumatologist, orthopedic surgeon, vascular surgeon, and even a rehab specialist. Each one offered well-intentioned therapies aimed at getting rid of the pain. Despite their efforts and interventions, I was left with intractable pain and nerve compression.

Years of physical therapy and emotional recovery opened my eyes to the reality of our medical system from a patient's perspective. As physicians, we simply take care of symptoms as they come up: painkillers for pain, sleeping pills for insomnia, anti-inflammatories for joint inflammation, and pills for the heartburn caused by the anti-inflammatory drugs. Surgical intervention comes with a myriad of risks and unforeseen side effects, such as my collapsed lung. Each action has a reaction. Some actions save lives, and I would not be here today without those necessary interventions. However, some others have far-reaching consequences that can be prevented. During my years of recovery, my symptoms were treated in isolation, but no one was there to integrate the symptoms or connect the dots.

Pain and terrifying dreams in which I relived the accident disrupted my nights. I woke up gasping for air in "fight-flight" reaction. The sleepless nights meant I overslept in the morning and woke too late to take my children to school. The medication made me feel drowsy, disconnected, and "foggy," and yet I needed pain relief. I struggled to control my symptoms so I could function as a mother and physician. I was caught in a vicious cycle of pain, insomnia, and fatigue, and being a physician did not help me break the cycle.

The reality of this situation came to a head when my then six-year-old daughter brought home a scrapbook called "Mommy and Me" for Mother's Day. The pictures she'd drawn were all of Mommy lying in bed with ice packs or heating pads, and the captions read, "My mommy is always tired" and "My mommy's neck hurts." I was shocked as I realized that this was how my daughter would remember me. I couldn't continue to watch passively from my bed with an exhausted body full of drugs, barely coping with the daily routine, as my children grew up. I had to break the vicious cycle of pain. That day, I decided to push back and find my way out: I had to reclaim my power, my health, and my personal and professional lives!

Delivering babies was no longer an option with my crushed shoulder. As a career transition, I enrolled in a mind-body course with Dr. Herbert Benson at Harvard University. He was at the cutting edge of research on the autonomic nervous system, the automatic "gas" and "brakes" in the body. Chronic exposure to stress hormones affects almost every system in our body and plays a key role in inflammation and illness. Through Dr. Benson's teachings, I realized that one of the most important factors for healing is learning to harness the immense potential of the mind and the nervous system. I learned I could get them working in unison to repair my body. And I did. What was supposed to be a career transition turned out to be the most radical transformation of my life!

I returned to Vancouver with renewed hope and determination. I researched and studied voraciously. I explored the role of chronic pain, anxiety, and trauma in healing. I learned that persistent pain and anxiety release a constant supply of stress hormones into the body and that nearly 75 percent of all visits to a doctor's office can be traced to the destructive effects of these hormones, which can disrupt sleep, cause fatigue, cause anxiety, and wreak havoc with the gut.[1] I had both chronic pain and anxiety from the mental trauma of the accident, and they continued to create major surges of stress hormones day and night.

Although the actual car accident had occurred only once, my brain replayed the memory like a broken tape, creating the same stress chemicals as it had at the moment of impact. I had lost so much ground, both physically and emotionally. The grief, fear, sadness, and loss were huge contributors to my stress response and were impeding my physical healing. I began to meditate, practice yoga, and heal both my mind and my gut, which had been wrecked by anti-inflammatory medications and painkillers.

Today, I help others to heal through principles of integrative medicine, which treats the body as a whole unit rather than as the sum of its parts. I knew other people could benefit from all I had learned and implemented in my life. *The Mind-Body Cure* is the culmination of my personal healing journey, my thirty years as a medical practitioner, and my research. It explains how and why chronic stress overwhelms and damages the body, and it reveals the practical tools I used to heal myself and the thousands of patients I have seen in my practice since that accident. Most importantly, the book highlights the profound role of our nervous system and its inextricable links to how and what we think. Therein lies the infinite and often untapped mine of possibilities for our health.

Introduction

MANY OF US are sick and tired. We run from one task to the next, checking off items on a to-do list. We eat snack food on the run. We get heartburn, so we take a pill and keep running. We end each day feeling exhausted, yet sleep does not come easily. We wake up feeling anxious. Chronic pain haunts us. We go on diets and gain weight. In numbers never seen before, we seek medical intervention for anxiety, depression, insomnia, gut problems, and immune diseases such as thyroid, joint, and skin problems. No matter what we do, the symptoms seem to get worse. Each prescription adds to the growing list of side effects.

Imagine if you no longer felt exhausted going from one errand to another. What if, after eating, you felt energized instead of fatigued or in discomfort? What if you woke up each morning feeling joyful, energetic, and healthy? What if you felt vibrant and in control of your symptoms and your health? All of this is possible. Many of our symptoms are connected. Our fatigue may be related to our insomnia, and our gut problems may put us at risk for autoimmune disease. Stress is a normal part of living, but when it gets out of control, it can negatively affect our health and well-being. Yet we can change that by learning to manage our unconscious reactions. Integrative medicine looks at how the body works as a unit and addresses the role of stress hormones as a major contributor to disease.

While our body can usually handle short-term stress, the effects of excessive, prolonged stress can lead to serious and life-threatening disease. Diabetes, depression, heart attacks, immune problems, respiratory problems, and even cancer are all associated with high levels of chronic stress. Data shows the deleterious effects of chronic inflammation resulting from years of stress on our brain and even our DNA. Globally, there is a trend to throw a "pill at every ill" without going to the root cause of the problem. If 75 percent of the symptoms that show up at doctors' offices can be attributed to chronic stress, then it makes sense to go to the root cause of the problem.

I was originally trained as a pharmacist and taught that drugs could treat most disease symptoms. Advil stops the pain. Pepto-Bismol helps settle upset stomachs. Vasotec lowers blood pressure. I soon realized these were stop-gap measures and I wanted to make more of a difference in people's lives, so I became a doctor. However, instead of filling prescriptions, I found myself writing them. With disease, doctors become proficient at "naming it, taming it, and blaming it." I recognized this type of medicine was very effective to manage symptoms but not the best approach to heal patients. Yet whenever I tried to use a holistic, whole-health approach, it resulted in longer wait times in my clinic.

I soon realized that the current medical system does not support physicians with the time, resources, or training required to address the root cause of the problem. We are so driven to cure a symptom with the latest technology or drug that we forget healing begins with the patient fully taking part in their care. But it wasn't until I experienced these deficits as a patient in the health-care system that I was really motivated to make integrative care the core of my practice as a doctor. What I learned from applying a mind-body approach to my own healing, and what I have subsequently confirmed while using an integrative approach with my patients, is that external solutions can help manage symptoms but long-lasting healing begins in the mind. Pain, anxiety, and fatigue are but a few of the symptoms of stress.

To ensure our survival as a species, the primitive human brain was designed to protect us at all costs: to scan for threats, avoid pain and seek pleasure, find the path of least resistance, and maximize efficiency. While humans and daily life have evolved over the millennia, our core preprogrammed neurological pathways remain the same. Though most of us no longer need to be wary of predators and fear for our lives daily, our quotidian fears and anxieties still travel the same pathways in the brain, provoking the same response as those original life-threatening situations. The constant triggering of this system creates disease.

Integrative medicine makes an important distinction between the mind and the brain. The brain—the collection of nerves and neurons centered in the skull that sends and receives chemical messages throughout the body—simply follows the program set out by our mind. The mind is the emotional, intellectual, and intuitive awareness that allows humans to feel, perceive, think, will, and especially reason. If our mind is our best friend and advocate, we are more resilient. If our mind is sabotaging us with beliefs of fear, alienation, or rejection, it becomes our biggest enemy.

When physicians do not investigate the multisystem causes of illness and tackle the true source of a symptom, we end up with patients who require more diagnostic tests and suffer side effects from drugs, both of which drive up the costs of health care. We just have to look at the staggering cost of health care in North America to see the impact of treating the symptom rather than the person. Instead, we need to change from this illness model to a wellness model. This is a radical shift in health care, and it is time for that change. All of us—doctors and patients—need to participate, and this book is an excellent start for those who want to take charge of their health and change their lives by changing their mindset.

In an illness model, doctors typically ask their patients, "How are you?" To which patients automatically reply, "I'm fine." This approach is easy, but it avoids any discussion of actual issues. What if doctors asked instead, "How did you sleep last night?" Invariably, we'd get a much more colorful answer that tells a deeper truth about how our patient feels. "My son has a cold and the new baby has been crying nonstop." Or "I can't stop thinking about when my heart will give out again." Suddenly, a concern replaces a standard answer, and doctors gain specific clues to support their patients' wellness. This is the first step in transitioning from the illness model to the wellness model of health.

In the past few years, I've furthered my own research and study in functional medicine and hormone health, become a Board Certified Menopause Clinician, and with Dr. Nishi Dhawan, co-founded the Westcoast Women's Clinic for Hormone Health, where we have provided holistic and integrative care to thousands of patients. In our practice, we promote a wellness model, and today I continue to pass on this knowledge and the tools I use to both my medical students and the community at large.

What you find in this book reflects my formal education, my research, and my clinical experience, including patient success stories, as well as my personal experience as a patient. You will learn why the autonomic nervous system (ANS) was the key to survival for our ancient ancestors and how this primitive defense system now works against us. You will learn how stress hormones attack the very organ that triggered their production: the brain.

A stressed brain triggers stress responses throughout the body, from our respiratory system to our gut, from our muscles to our immune system. The result is illness and disease throughout the body. The first eight chapters of the book describe how stress affects each of our body systems and the types of damage that result. Each of those chapters also explains how to cultivate a health mindset and provides practical tools that engage the mind and use it to short-circuit our stress response and allow the body to heal. The final chapter brings together seven practical tools in one place, providing a whole-body REFRAME toolkit to beat chronic stress. I firmly believe that all our body systems are interrelated. When we address the root cause of illness—the stress in our mind, our brain, and our body—we begin to heal and set the foundation for long-lasting health.

My purpose in this book is not to discredit modern medical practice, nor is it to discount the role of diet, genetics, and other factors in disease. We can still address all these elements. But simple, realistic changes to mindset and lifestyle can bring positive changes to your health right now. I want to give you the tools to bring accountability for health into your own hands. I want you to understand how chronic emotional stress is connected to physical symptoms. And more importantly, I want you to learn why it is important to regulate your emotions so that your nervous system works for you and not against you.

When I now think back to my accident, I believe something phenomenal came out of something terrible. By learning to regulate my nervous system, I transformed my personal health. I reprogrammed my mind to obtain a better response in the body. As a physician, I became better equipped to optimize health for others, and I have dramatically changed the way I practice medicine. My patients heal! I feel compelled to share my message with others, and I hope this book is the start of your own health journey. What you learn will ask you to acknowledge the inner dialogue and embedded beliefs that dictate how you make decisions for your health. Be prepared to make up your mind to create a healthier body! Are you ready to get started?

1.

Mind Your Mind

The greatest weapon against stress is our ability to choose one thought over another.
William James

SELF-ASSESSMENT

Mental or emotional health refers to overall psychological well-being and the ability to control thoughts, feelings, and behaviors. Individuals who cope with stress more effectively and better manage anger, fear, and negative emotions tend to be healthier. People who struggle with mental or emotional health may need to improve the tools and skills needed to effectively deal with stress. They often feel stuck in life.

Do you:

- believe that you have little to no control over health?

- constantly criticize yourself and have a negative inner dialogue?

- have mood swings or react with angry outbursts?

- look after others but have difficulty with self-care?

- take criticism harshly or often feel rejected?

- slip into negative thought patterns such as "not enoughness"?

- have trouble feeling motivated and excited about life?

- fear making mistakes and have the need to be perfect?

- struggle with minor daily stressors, such as traffic, while others cope and thrive?

- worry excessively about health?

- blame others or circumstances when you feel poorly?

We start with the mind because that is ultimately where we make choices and decisions that affect our health, sometimes consciously and more often unconsciously. How we perceive the world is more a reflection of our beliefs and thoughts and less about the reality that surrounds us. Many books discuss the connection between our mind and our body, but many of them miss the very important connection between our mind and our brain, specifically the intricate and close association of our thoughts to our body's autonomous regulation centers. We can allow our negative thoughts to run automatically, signaling our brain to constantly release stress hormones that ultimately create disease. Alternatively, we can control our thoughts, choose our beliefs, and consciously affect our brain, reducing and eliminating stress and disease. Thus, we start our exploration of the mind-brain-body connection with an exploration of the mind.

MIND MATTERS

Most people use the terms "mind" and "brain" interchangeably. In fact, they are two related but very distinct entities. Our brain is an amazing organ with a definite shape, size, and function. It is three pounds of convoluted gray and white matter that looks like tofu and represents millions of nerve cells, nerves, and blood vessels. Humans used to think that only our species had a brain. We now know that many other species, from fruit flies to blue whales, have some kind of brain and nervous system to run their body. We also know that the shape and size of the human brain have changed over the millennia we have walked on Earth. For example, the frontal lobe of the modern human's brain is remarkably larger and more developed than that of a Neanderthal human. Today, we view the brain as the control center for all our body's actions. For example, when you accidentally touch a hot stove, the pain signals are communicated within a millisecond to the brain, you pull your hand away quickly, and further damage is controlled.

Our mind is more difficult to define because it is abstract. While most living things have a brain, the mind is harder to measure in other species. It is made up of concepts, beliefs, and individual perceptions based on our memories and experiences. The mind can evaluate situations, process information, and make decisions consciously or subconsciously. How do we x-ray someone's mind? What does it look like? How big is it? Where is it located? The mind is a function of the brain but does not necessarily reside in the brain; the mind is the sense of awareness, consciousness, and intelligence that we all have. For example, imagine you say something on a whim that upsets someone, and you stop and think to yourself, "Why the heck did I say that?"

Who is the thinker doing that reflective thinking? The observer of all the narration and thoughts that go on in the brain is the conscious mind, and the conscious mind is exclusive to humans (at least we used to presume it was).

In the 1800s, many intellectuals discussed whether specific areas of the brain controlled different parts and functions of the body, or if the whole brain integrating all of its various parts affected the entire body. A lot of discussion and research in this area was fueled by the case of Phineas Gage,[1] a railroad foreman who suffered a brain injury in 1848. While he was directing a crew blasting rock to level the railbed, an iron rod pierced his skull on the left side just forward of the jaw, passed behind his left eye and through the left side of his brain, and then exited through the top of his skull. Extraordinarily, the young man's life was spared. Before his head injury, Gage was described by people who knew him as a kind, sober, compassionate, moral, and friendly young man. After the accident, his friends and family observed a very different personality. He drank and became aggressive; he used profane language and became a belligerent jerk to all who came in contact with him. The man they once knew was gone. What is more surprising is that Gage recognized he was drastically different—he had an awareness and memory of his previous self—but could not control his behavior.

Scientists began to explore whether personality lives in the prefrontal cortex, the part of Gage's brain that was pierced by the rod. Over a century passed before technology had developed enough that neuroscience could map out areas in the brain responsible for functions such as speech, physical movement, cognition, and memory storage. Scientists learned that the prefrontal cortex controls higher decision-making, personality traits, and judgment but not the awareness of self. Gage lost his inhibitions and his ability to filter emotions of right and wrong. He lost various personality traits, but the question remained whether he also lost his mind. Who was the observer in Gage's brain that was "aware" he was behaving or thinking differently than before the accident?

The Mind as Distinct from the Brain

Mapping out our brain function has been fairly straightforward. Over the years, researchers have stimulated parts of the brain and looked for corresponding movement in the body so that we now have a concrete map of what areas in the brain control the many functions of our body, such as speech, hearing, sight, movement, and balance. This map remains fairly consistent from one human brain to another. Mapping mind function has been much more challenging, because there appears to be no rhyme or reason to the way people behave, and depending on whom you ask, you will get a variety of answers as to how the brain and mind are related.

Scientists do seem to agree on one thing: humans possess a trait called metacognition, the ability to have an awareness and understanding of our own thought processes. In other words, we think about thinking. We can use this power to be more precise about what, how, and why we think a certain way to optimize our behavior, performance, and understanding, which is why neuroscientists, psychologists, and psychiatrists continue to try to unravel the complexities of the human mind—each of them coming at these questions from a different perspective.

Neurologists are medical doctors who study the brain, nerves, and nervous systems. Most of them seem to have a very definite answer for how the mind and the brain are related. The mind is a function of the brain, of course! A functioning brain is identical to a conscious mind, they explain, and mind expression is science in its highest form. With no brain, there would be no mind. Therefore, they contend that consciousness is nothing more than the ability of our brain to acquire information (i.e., awake state), understand the content of that information, and then store and retrieve information from our memory. For example, a patient who suffers a massive stroke is no longer conscious but their brain is working. We know this because their heart, lungs, gut, and circulation all continue to work despite the patient's lack of consciousness. But what about the mind? We don't know. The patient is unconscious or sometimes in a coma. We do not have the means to see if their mind is functioning; however, if we develop more sophisticated means of measuring thought, perhaps this will become more precise.

Psychologists study human behavior and they seem to hold a very "dualistic" theory. They argue that the mind and the brain are two distinct entities, that many people have a fully functioning brain and are awake but "lose or disconnect from their mind." That is, though people have the ability to feel empathy and compassion, they may become so self-absorbed that these functions of the mind are blunted and their brain automatically runs their bodily functions. Sometimes people who have experienced trauma or adversity disconnect from the memory by not engaging with the conscious mind, as it causes pain and suffering. Thus, they function physically but disconnected from the mind. They may choose to use alcohol or drugs or food to numb the memories that the mind keeps bringing up.

Most psychologists maintain the mind has a conscious and a subconscious component. They state that we spend much of our childhood or formative years collecting information on speech and behavior by observing and mimicking those around us, and we lock in these unprocessed memories, associated emotions, and patterns for future reference. This embedded program is often what we use as our reference point for the rest of our lives. It becomes our subconscious mind. It is what forms the basis of construct or mindset, which we will explore later. In contrast, our conscious mind is the objective perspective of the mind that identifies information, compares and analyzes it with known information, and decides what to do.

Psychiatrists are medical doctors trained to deal with mental illnesses such as depression, schizophrenia, and bipolar disorders, and they are able to prescribe medications as well as psychotherapy. They generally consider impairments in the biochemistry or anatomy of the brain as the reason for mental illness. They agree that psychosocial aspects of childhood, genetics, and experienced trauma play a role in people's behavior. Many studies show that psychosis and bipolar disorders are brain disorders that result from an imbalance of chemicals in the brain and manifest as aberrations in thought, mood, cognition, and behavior.[2] Psychiatrists treat disorders of the mind with both behavior psychotherapy and medications. Although they seem to distinguish between mind and brain, they see the mind as a complex matrix of many factors that come into play, including biochemical or anatomical problems of the brain.

Mind dualists such as psychologists and psychiatrists view the subconscious mind as the backdrop against which we carry out all our conscious functions of memory, communication, learning, and applying information. It influences our entire life in ways we don't always comprehend. We make choices, judgments, and decisions unaware that our subconscious mind is in control of our habits and automatic behaviors. The world's most well-known and most controversial psychoanalyst, Sigmund Freud, used an iceberg to illustrate this idea. He said we experience or "see" only the uppermost 10 percent of an iceberg rising above the water's surface. This part of the iceberg is our conscious mind. The remaining 90 percent of the iceberg, the subconscious, lies beneath the waves and is imperceptible.[3] While the conscious mind might assume it's directing the iceberg, in reality the waves and currents acting on our subconscious are the true navigators.

Finally, spiritual scholars claim the mind is our soul—a moral and emotional guiding force that examines universal truths—and belongs to the conscious spiritual realm. Those who have learned to align with this way of thinking feel a profound and conscious connection to a higher power. They remain dualists because they find it difficult or impossible to accept that brain function alone can explain consciousness. That is, they maintain that even after all the specialized cells of the brain have fired, all the associated chemical messages have been sent and received, and we have performed complex tasks, something is missing. Spiritual scholars maintain that a universal or cosmic consciousness controls these effects and not just biology, physics, and chemistry.

Delving into the complex field of mind science is an evolving process and we may never agree on one definition. As a physician, I have seen the powerful effect of thoughts and beliefs on behavior, choices, and health outcomes. I recognize that connecting our mind to our body is vitally important if we want to make changes in our biology. As a patient, I can say that a "mind shift" had to occur for me to make a mental leap from an illness to a wellness mindset, and it began with changing my thoughts, beliefs, inner dialogue, and behavior.

For now, the mystery of the mind continues to elude us. New technology and advanced diagnostics have made it possible to use functional magnetic resonance imaging (fMRI) machines to measure emotions as millions of nerve impulses being transmitted and received by cells throughout the body. This specialized neuroimaging allows us to see areas in the brain light up when thought alone directs blood flow there. By looking at patterns across hundreds of images, scientists can diagnose emotions of the brain. We can tell when someone is angry, focused on a task, in love, or depressed. This technology will be useful in diagnosing mental illnesses and thought patterns associated with physical disease. Soon enough we will also be able to measure visceral body functions such as blood flow to the gut by examining conscious thought. As we see these connections between our thoughts and their physical manifestations in the body, we are getting closer to understanding how we might use the mind to change or mediate these impulses.

The Multidimensional Mind

One of the best explanations of the mind, in my opinion, comes from comparing research done by psychologists with the experience of spiritual scholars who realize that the mind is not a single physical construct but a multidimensional "mental body." This mind definition comprises four dimensions: intelligence, practical knowledge, body memory, and consciousness.

Intelligence refers to our concrete memory and knowledge. This is similar to reading a manual about how to drive a car without actually driving the car. It is knowledge without practical experience. The second dimension refers to mind as our practical knowledge, how we apply our intelligence. This is like when you finally get in a car and drive. The experience is very different from just reading about it, which is why many people pass the written driving exam but fail the practical driving test. So it is with the mind. Many people have read books about mind-body medicine and they recognize there is a connection, but they have not yet experienced it or been able to apply the knowledge because they haven't mastered the techniques or applied them to their health.

The third dimension is body memory, which incorporates the belief that every cell in our body has a mind. We have traditionally confined the "mind" to our head and brain, but the work of cell biologist Dr. Bruce Lipton shows that all cells hold memory and can respond to their environment.[4] For example, our cells change their behavior and genetic characteristics depending on whether our thoughts are negative or positive. His research reveals that we should view cell membranes rather than the DNA in the cell as "mini" brains. We also know that certain cells carry memory of a skill or a trauma. For example, placing the fingers of a pianist with Alzheimer's disease or dementia on a keyboard can elicit a physical response by the finger muscles allowing them to play music. Similarly, a muscle that was once injured can go into spasm just by thinking about the events that precipitated the injury. The fourth dimension, consciousness, is untarnished by memory, conditioning, or bias. This is the pure form of innate intelligence, our ability to function with conscience, universal truths, and divine knowledge that take the mind into a spiritual dimension that many call the soul.

If we consider the mind from this multidimensional perspective, we see that the mind lives nowhere. Rather, it exists everywhere, lives throughout our body, and is fundamental to our unique individual experiences. Perhaps as more sophisticated tools for mind mapping become available, we will find better ways to quantify or understand the human mind. Until then, I think it's best to have an open view of what we think of as the human mind. My opinion is that our mind is a field of potential energy that may be connected to a universal field of consciousness, but I don't expect others to hold the same view. For the purposes of this book, it is enough to consider that our mind is separate from our brain and that it has the ability to influence the brain, both consciously and subconsciously.

UNDERSTANDING MINDSET

We have examined the mind and its various dimensions. We understand that the brain is constantly generating thoughts and random observations that are fleeting. A mindset is a specific lens or frame of mind that orients us to a particular set of associations and expectations; it is our unique view of the world.[5] It runs our body "automatically," as if on autopilot. Our mindset can be influenced by our conscious mind, our subconscious mind, or a combination of the two. As we've seen, psychologists believe that our subconscious mind forms the backdrop to most of our thinking. Our experiences with things and people in our early life and the emotions and meaning we associate with those experiences are stored in our subconscious and form the basis of our mindset. To change your mind in an instant is easy, but to change your mindset requires more work and this is the premise of creating health.

Some of us naturally gloss over the negative and see everything through rose-colored glasses, whereas some of us store and amplify negative experiences. For example, adverse childhood experiences often negatively influence our mindset.[6] While it intrigues me whether optimism and pessimism are inherited traits or acquired, our subconsciously stored memories cause us to view life experiences with a pre-set lens. This subconscious program contains paths of least resistance, familiar outcomes, and often fear-based behaviors. And while this automatic mechanism can help us operate efficiently for repetitive tasks, allowing our subconscious pathways to run our entire life is problematic if we have downloaded bad habits or conditioned ourselves to less-than-optimal health. Ideally, it would be wonderful if we could simply have a mindset that was automatically set to default to healthy behaviors.

Although many of us have good intentions when it comes to our health, we easily fall back on automatic habits and become derailed when we don't involve our conscious mind. And if our subconscious lens magnifies negative experiences, we may even look for negative experiences to reinforce what is pre-set, thereby sabotaging our best efforts to make change. It requires awareness, effort, intention, and repetition to transform poor habits into good habits. I know from my own practice that some people run an automatic program of health and wellness and overcome obstacles more easily than those who have a mindset of blame, shame, guilt, or being a victim. Others continually run into challenges, oblivious to the automatic expectations they have set up for themselves. The bottom line is that our mind can make us sick or our mind can manufacture health. Thus, we must choose carefully and consciously what program we want running our body automatically (subconsciously)!

How Mindset Affects Our Health

I often use the analogy of modern-day computers to describe the mind-brain-body connection. I compare the mind to a programmer who builds a software program, the brain to the computer that runs the software program, and the body to the display screen or monitor on which the program is shown. As physicians, we often look just at the display screen when we measure symptoms (blood pressure, heart rate, gut function, or even blood tests). We often prescribe drugs or order tests based on what we find there (the physical symptoms) without really going deeper into which "program" that particular body is playing. If mindset is the software program being played by the computer, it often needs "upgrades and updates" and sometimes needs to be replaced completely. A new program results in a whole new set of information being displayed on the monitor. When it comes to the software program—our mindset—we have control over the version we choose.

➤ Growth Mindset versus Fixed Mindset
In her book *Mindset: The New Psychology of Success*, researcher Carol Dweck showed that mindset—whether growth or fixed— was a profound determinant of a person's performance.[7] She defined people who believe their success is based on innate ability as having a fixed mindset; that is, they think they are born with a certain amount of intelligence and talent and that's that. Either they know something or they don't. Those who believe their success is based on hard work, learning, training, and doggedness, she defined as having a growth mindset. If they don't succeed at something the first time, they think that hard work and learning will allow them to master it. Many different cultures value diligent work, and we know that working hard (and working smart) is a great way to achieve our goals. Yet we also believe people have innate natural talents that give them an advantage.

For example, we look at people like Albert Einstein or Michael Jordan and see that their natural talents gave them both success and notability. However, their inherent talent was not the only quality they had. Dweck points out that talent alone would not have been enough. Imagine if Einstein had written the theory of relativity and then just kicked back and drunk lemonade! The fact he persisted and continued to create world-changing theories shows he was hungry for knowledge and disciplined enough to continue his research. This made him one of the most revered physicists in history. In the same way, what if Michael Jordan had hooped a few basketballs with precision and then quit just to lie around reveling in his glory? Would we remember him today? Absolutely not. Both men had more than incredible natural talent. They had other qualities in common, such as persistence, curiosity, and grit. They continued to practice and hone their skill and talent. Incredible natural talent combined with a mindset for improvement and effort produced epic results.

We can apply this mindset theory to our health. Believing in our ability to change our life is a key feature of a growth mindset, compared with assuming we possess immutable characteristics with a fixed mindset. In clinical practice, I have witnessed various patterns of mindset when treating patients over the years. I refer to those patients as having a health mindset versus an illness mindset. When we believe inherently that our mindset (software program) is not etched in stone, we can "upgrade" and "update" the version of software that our brain is playing so we get better results. Those results are displayed by the body. The programmer (our conscious mind) is key when it comes to starting this process.

➤ Health Mindset

People with a health mindset trust that they have some control over their health outcomes. They are willing to learn about health, adopt new behaviors, and commit to making a change with the confidence that it will produce change. In fact, some of these people have such faith in self-healing they have spontaneously healed themselves or responded to placebos alone.

People with a growth mindset know that putting in more time and effort can make them smarter, more intelligent, and talented. Those with a health mindset are healthier individuals! Why? Because they formed subconscious beliefs in their childhood that they could control their health—or they learned later in life that they could control their choices in health—and through practice and effort, they achieve better outcomes. Remember the saying, "Hard work beats talent if talent doesn't work hard." If we want to be healthy, we must put in the effort to form healthy habits of thinking, living, and doing.

A health mindset doesn't always come naturally, but once we understand that our beliefs influence our body at a cellular level, we can learn and develop the ability to improve our health outcomes. In fact, we have an incredible influence over our health skills and abilities, far more influence than we know. Except for extremely rare cases of strong genetics, our genes define only a limited amount for us.

➤ Illness Mindset

People with a fixed mindset assume that ability and understanding are concrete and fixed, so they don't try to change. They often assume that their DNA is their destiny—they were either born with health or they weren't—and therefore believe they don't have control over their health outcomes. This "what's the point?" attitude to changing behaviors for health is a form of illness mindset. A defeatist attitude, we now know, can lead to disease and even failed treatments. In other words, fixed-mindset individuals sabotage themselves before they even start. They don't commit to changing their lifestyle because they have a core belief that nothing will help.

Why does nothing work on those patients? It's called the "nocebo" effect. Individuals contribute to their illness by subconsciously creating chemicals of self-destruction. They convince themselves that nothing will work, so it often doesn't. How many times have people with cancer learned they have six months to live, and they do, while others refuse to be boxed in and outlive their disease or even beat cancer?

The main differences between the two mindsets of health and illness are our belief in the permanence of intelligence about our health state, our ability to adapt to any change in environment, and the knowledge that our circumstances do not define us. People with a health mindset are open to growth and change with opportunities for improvement. They can adapt to new information and adopt new behaviors; they are more resilient. In these individuals, we can update the software program that runs the body.

Case Study: Jane and Carol

In my family practice many years ago, two unrelated patients, Jane and Carol, were diagnosed with breast cancer within a few weeks of each other. They were only a few years apart in age. Their biopsy results were coincidentally identical on the pathology report, so I referred them both to a well-known cancer specialist in the area. He ended up seeing them a few weeks apart.

Carol was a happy-go-lucky, charming, and no-nonsense woman who was very proactive about her health. I explained the report of cancer; she appeared surprised at the diagnosis. Yet Carol calmly asked a few questions and then responded, "Doctor, just do whatever you need to do to get this thing out of me. I have travel plans and grandchildren to care for." On the way out, she asked if I could recommend some good reading resources.

When I called Jane in to inform her of the diagnosis, she reacted in a state of panic before I could give her all the information. She had lost an aunt to breast cancer many years earlier and watched her die. No amount of reassurance and education about new treatments would convince Jane that she would not necessarily have the same outcome as her aunt. It took a lot of time to calm her down so I could explain the next steps.

Shortly after the initial visit, both Carol and Jane required the same surgery, which the same surgeon performed. The same oncologist at the same hospital prescribed the same chemotherapy and radiation protocol. Since the pathology report was the same, they received the same course of medical treatment.

Due to her anxious mood, I referred Jane for counseling and a cancer support group. Counselors reported that Jane lived with the fear of pain and death and had little faith in herself or the medical system. Her anxiety became so severe, I also had to prescribe sleeping pills and anxiety medication. Occasionally, the anxiety escalated to debilitating panic attacks. She rarely left her house except to attend medical appointments. Jane cut herself off from friends and stopped going to church.

It's important to recognize that having anxiety isn't "wrong" or "bad." Anxiety is energy, and it is up to us how we channel that energy. In Jane's case, anxiety was a maladaptive emotion that made her body sick. Carol chose to channel her "anxious" energy into constructive behavior to keep herself motivated toward her goals of traveling and spending time with her grandchildren.

The oncologist and I had discussions about Jane's lack of response to cancer treatment, the severe side effects, and the poor prognosis she faced. Carol also had side effects of chemo and many rough days, but her follow-up reports were excellent. The staggering difference perplexed me. Why were these two women responding so differently to the same treatment when surgery had confirmed identical pathology? Had I missed something? I second-guessed myself and reviewed both files after work one day, trying to find a reason why one patient was declining day by day and the other patient was improving.

Sadly, Jane continued to get sicker. Her cancer spread to other organs including her brain, and she lost her battle with cancer after eighteen months of treatment. For Jane, it had truly been a "battle." She was angry and scared and saw her cancer as the enemy.

Carol had a fairly good recovery despite the awful side effects. When she lost all her hair, she went out and bought several wigs and called them funny names. Marilyn Monroe was her blond wig. A dark brown wig with a whitish streak she called "Roadkill." Carol kept up a good front of humor and she remained grateful for each day; she saw her cancer as a "gift" to remind her to live each day to the fullest. Today, Carol is still alive and cancer-free, and I receive occasional cards and messages from her. She went on a cruise and has made countless memories with her grandchildren.

These two patient interactions forced me to consider the stark difference in their attitude and mindset. Jane had accepted defeat before she began the fight. She feared death far more than she trusted herself and the medical system. Jane truly believed the cancer would kill her, and it did. She had fixed beliefs of an illness mindset and no one had the power to change her beliefs. That is the profound power of the "nocebo" effect.

While the benefits of cultivating a health mindset are desirable, just thinking about it and "espousing" it are not enough. "Think healthy thoughts and you will be healthy," many self-help books profess. It may be a step in the right direction, but positive thinking backed by a health mindset and applied ability—effort and practice—guarantee better outcomes. The positive knowledge and dialogue have to become a part of the subconscious narrative; we must have faith that we are a part of our healing and that healing begins inside. And we must act on that belief.

HOW TO CULTIVATE A HEALTH MINDSET

As a physician, I have learned to recognize the qualities that are a common denominator for health when assessing patients. Individuals with a health mindset see health obstacles as challenges and learn how to navigate them by asking questions and staying open, curious, and informed. They are compassionate and kind toward themselves. They work harder and smarter than other patients because they know they are worth it and are confident about being in charge of their health.

They show their vulnerability and ask for help when needed. They display a can-do attitude. They step outside their comfort zone to get the health outcomes they need and want. They see a future for themselves and have cultivated family or friend support systems. They have purpose and want to live better. Those with a health mindset are more likely to see diagnosis of an illness as a challenge to overcome and seek opportunities to improve their coping skills and enhance their knowledge. They often reframe their adverse experience as a "gift" rather than a curse. It helps if they are lighthearted and possess humor. The ability to laugh at themselves or at life and realize being healthy doesn't have to be a serious business goes a long way.

In my practice, I recall a patient who had a terrible car accident, an athletic student who suffered multiple injuries including damage to the spinal cord. Doctors said he would never walk again. He took this as a challenge and proved them wrong. He was walking in less than a year; through sheer grit and determination, he achieved what doctors considered medically impossible. There are hundreds of cases where patients have gone against the odds to prove the medical establishment wrong for boxing them in. If we examined their pre-sickness personality, we would find they had a health mindset before they became ill. They had a permanent belief, an inner wisdom, an ability to trust that they had options, and their ability to respond was "unlimited" even if their circumstances were limited. To cultivate healing, I urge my patients to be active participants in their healing and hold on to their power by being responsible and accountable for their choices. It's a lesson I had to learn firsthand.

➤ My Story

After my accident, I remained in a holding pattern of physical and emotional pain for quite some time, for several reasons. I had developed an inner dialogue of being a "victim." I blamed the driver: "He should have been watching." I blamed myself: "I could have taken a different route home." Sometimes I pitied myself because I felt it was unfair the accident happened to me. Losing my baby made me upset, sad, and frustrated—I knew I was in no shape to have more children in my condition and I wasn't getting any younger, but I wanted a bigger family. I developed terrible insomnia, mostly because of chronic physical pain and nightmares of the accident. This left me with severe fatigue, which was often debilitating.

I was led to conclude the only answer to my situation was more drugs and more surgeries, yet neither appealed to me. By that time, I had tried many different medications, received several injections, done a variety of physical therapies, and even undergone multiple surgeries. Nothing had provided sustained relief for the chronic pain. Looking back, I now see that I was in an illness mindset because I felt hopeless: nothing had worked, and as a result, I believed there was no end in sight. I also believed I didn't have the power to change my outcome, that I was a victim of my circumstances and pain and loss, that I just had to put up with it. And being a physician compounded the problem, because I often felt that if I couldn't heal myself, how could I expect to help others.

My first step to healing was starting to become aware of my "self," especially the thoughts that were not serving me well. I began to notice the repeated patterns of negative thoughts and make a conscious effort to think more positively. For example, instead of mourning the loss of my unborn child, I began to focus on the two beautiful children already in my life. Instead of seeing the loss of my career delivering babies as a failure, I began to focus on what possibilities were going to come from this situation someday. Instead of resenting the physical pain in my body, I began to see it as telling me to pay more attention to self-care and be more kind and compassionate to myself. Reframing my thoughts and making that change to a new mindset for healing took awareness, insight, energy, and time, but it was the best prescription I have ever filled.

Upgrade Your Inner Dialogue

Look within and take an honest inventory of your current beliefs to cultivate self-awareness. Perhaps you have negative subconscious thoughts or you run automatic self-limiting programs. Perhaps you have raw untapped potential that you need to develop. Gather feedback from trusted friends and family about your unique strengths and weaknesses (like a business "strengths, weaknesses, opportunities, and threats" or SWOT analysis). If your self-talk is negative, take steps to upgrade your inner dialogue using the stop, observe, detach, affirm (SODA) technique.

➤ Stop, Observe, Detach, Affirm

The SODA technique, often used by cognitive behavioral therapists, is a way to consciously reframe a situation. It's especially useful when your thinking patterns are stuck on repeat and you need to hit pause so you can take a step back and assess what's going on. I originally learned this technique when I took a course with integrative medicine advocate Deepak Chopra, and I have found it helpful for both myself and my patients. I highly recommend this as your first step in cultivating a health mindset.

- *Stop* refers to our ability to gain control over our thoughts. Be the mind that does the thinking.

- *Observe* refers to metacognition, your mind witnessing your thoughts and emotions as a third party without judgment or action.

- *Detach* means to abandon negative, automatic, fear-based pathways once you recognize them.

- *Affirm* means to create another, positive thought so it can replace the automatic negative thought.

When trauma interferes in our lives, we have the power to become stronger and better. We need to understand how to do that, use the right tools, and seek support. As a physician, I urge you to consciously and objectively evaluate your mindset. If you are inclined to sit back and let someone fix you, acknowledge that. But to heal, you will need to cultivate a health mindset. Learn to take responsibility. Research, participate, and contribute to creating ways to fix the problem. Believe that you can help fix the situation. If you are willing to put in the time and effort, developing a health mindset is possible.

$$\longleftrightarrow$$

TRY THESE ADDITIONAL STEPS to master your health mindset.

➤ Surround Yourself with Positive Role Models of Health
It is much easier to adopt a health mindset when you see it working for others, so look around you and observe the behavior of

healthy people. Meet people who have learned to overcome their health obstacles. Join support groups if that is helpful. Read books that encourage and inspire you in your journey. Listen to podcasts or watch videos on how others have navigated the transition from illness to health. Then emulate these individuals who possess a health mindset, even if you have to "fake it until you make it" when you start.

➤ Be Passionate

Give yourself a reason or a set of reasons to be passionate about pursuing a health mindset. For example, remember a time when you felt vibrant and healthy and dwell on that image with all your senses. Feel that strength. When passion fuels our goals, we align our body, heart, and head and feel content, which makes it easy to do what we love. Passion, purpose, and perspective help motivate us for more self-improvement.

➤ Be Persistent

It takes determination and hard work to reprogram a mindset. Acknowledge that you will need to navigate obstacles and be tenacious enough to do so. Prepare for challenges by setting and writing down interim goals for yourself. If or when you slip back into old thought patterns and behaviors, gently and consciously bring your attention back to your new program and to one of your interim goals. Use the time just before you go to sleep to think of all the things you are thankful for. Think about the gains you've made to help you stay motivated and cultivate persistence.

➤ Practice Self-Compassion and Kindness

This is the cornerstone of mastering a health mindset. Unconditionally accepting ourselves, knowing we are resourceful, knowing we are imperfectly perfect and inherently good, and knowing we are never alone are vital beliefs to create the foundation of self-trust. Instead of saying, "I am never going to get better," focus on what you are doing to heal and tell yourself, "I am getting better every day." Say these words out loud to make them real and powerful. If you occasionally slip into your old illness mindset with a negative comment or if you eat some junk food or don't make time for exercise from time to time, be gentle and forgive yourself. Vow to try harder next time and move on!

Don't just take my word for it: research shows that self-forgiveness is associated with both mental and physical health. In a review of many major studies involving almost 18,000 participants, researchers found a robust correlation between self-forgiveness and psychological well-being.[8]

➤ Be Open and Curious

Health and wellness are broad topics. Gaining knowledge and information about your illness is important, but try not to become consumed with the details. Be willing to ask questions to enhance your current knowledge. You don't have to be an instant expert in any one subject, but pay more attention to how you could be a more active participant in your health care. Asking questions and actively listening to answers improves results.

➤ Practice Mindfulness

"Mindfulness is a state of active, open attention in the present. When you are mindful you observe your thoughts and feelings from a distance, without judging them good or bad. Mindfulness means living in the moment and awakening to experience."[9] Bringing your attention to the present moment and remaining fully in the "now" is the foundation of mindfulness, and it's a great way to pause the brain's automatic playback loop of past fears and failures. Use all your senses to register what you are doing at that moment, whether it is breathing, eating, buying groceries, etc. Enlisting the senses to hyperfocus on something you can touch, smell, or hear magically turns off the stress response.

Try doing this with a raisin (or an almond). Begin by observing it visually. Really notice how wrinkled it is. Look closely at the color: how dark brown it is, how it has a slightly frosty tinge. Now pick it up. Touch all the ridges and squeeze it gently to test its consistency. Close your eyes and explore it with your fingers, and then lightly place it on your tongue. Feel the ridges on the raisin and notice how it makes contact with your palate, cheeks, or gums. Now gently bite into the raisin and notice the soft flesh in your mouth, savor the sweetness. Feel grateful for having this experience and being able to fully enjoy the raisin before you swallow it.

Being mindful is having a state of active, open attention in the present moment while observing your thoughts and feelings without judgment. A heightened sense of awareness during mindfulness, using all your senses, allows you to re-create the memory of the raisin later without actually eating one. Your brain registers this experience so deeply on a multisensory level that when you recall it, your body will produce the same chemicals as if there were a raisin on your tongue. The same applies to your health. When you are in an illness mindset or your stress level is rising, you can slow down, be mindful, and allow your mind to re-create the memory of health and positivity.

The Benefits of a Healthy Mindset

When we move from simply knowing about health to actively cultivating a health mindset, our thoughts, actions, and feelings change. We form a habit of self-approval rather than seeking outside validation. We become more resilient. We become more open to learning from others and from our own mistakes, and we become more confident in our abilities to persevere when challenged and to develop strategies that support our health. Our attitude adjustment is our responsibility and no one else can do that for us.

Challenging your automatic thoughts and learning to reframe situations and view them in different ways creates new neural networks and allows you to manage your own health. By mastering the tools that create a health mindset, you can ensure an inner dialogue that is pro health rather than pro disease. Remember that thinking positive thoughts is not enough; only by trusting at a deep core level that there will be positive outcomes will our brain translate this message to all the cells in the body. This is the fundamental basis for long-term physical health, vitality, and longevity because positive thought patterns lead to healthy choices in behavior, which then become traits, and eventually turn into habits, which form the basis of what becomes your health-conscious personality.

Having a health mindset allows you to set specific, realistic health goals and achieve them. Instead of committing to "follow a healthy diet," you are more likely to succeed if you write down your intention to "eat a boiled egg, one cup of berries, and one cup of oatmeal with shredded coconut for breakfast." Having a tangible, specific, and doable goal engages your conscious brain and gives you a precise target to follow through on. Similarly, if you want to lose weight, engage your health mindset and declare, "I have confidence in my ability to walk briskly for at least thirty minutes daily, then add thirty sit-ups before I go to bed."

In my own recovery, I initially underestimated the power of the mind, the inner dialogue, and the role of stress hormones on inflammation and healing. Healing does not occur overnight, and my journey continues today. I still occasionally get flare-ups of neck pain while doing certain activities, but I am better at body and mind awareness and can recalibrate faster. I still get the occasional terrifying dream of the accident, but I can recover much more quickly and not let it affect my day.

The difference is that the memory of the accident no longer triggers visceral anxiety and panic or emotions. More importantly, my perception (my story) has shifted from "Why did this happen to me?" to "It could have been much worse; I am alive and well now." I have taken full responsibility for my pain and recovery rather than staying in victim mode. I have practiced forgiveness for the driver and for myself. I have become a better physician as I view treatment and health care differently. I view the accident and all I have become as a gift to live a new and better life.

CONCLUSION

As humans, we are products of what we think, believe, and feel—and the mind rather than the brain is at the center of these. Thoughts are the language of the mind. Established thoughts become beliefs, and they are the language of our mindset and the way we see the world. Feelings are the language of the body. To change how we feel, we must change our thoughts and beliefs.

Our mind manufactures 50,000 to 60,000 thoughts per day! Many of those are automatic responses embedded in our subconscious and they underlie our belief systems and our mindset. Think about that for a minute. If we could consciously harness all of those thoughts for health, just think how powerful that could be. The key to healing illness rests on staying alert and observing our automatic thoughts, and if these are negative, then we need to actively create new, better thoughts that serve our body. When repeated, virtually experienced, and "felt," these beliefs become embedded in our subconscious mind and become our new automatic thoughts. This is the ultimate "shift" that occurs in mindset and sets us in motion toward healing or better health.

2.

Mind
Your Brain

*The brain is a world consisting of a
number of unexplored continents and
great stretches of unknown territory.*
Santiago Ramón y Cajal

SELF-ASSESSMENT

Our brain is designed to be efficient and to automatically stream-line the activities of daily life, especially repetitive ones. We become creatures of habit: doing the same things, buying the same food, cooking the same way, and even sitting at the same seat every day. We are unaware that our brain is running things automatically with no conscious input.

Do you:

· have a morning routine (for example, get up, go to the toilet, prepare your coffee ...)?

· have a favorite mug for your coffee or tea?

· sit in the same seat at the table, at the movies, or on the bus?

- walk into the kitchen and automatically open the fridge door?

- eat reflexively when you see food ads?

- go to familiar Internet or YouTube sites?

- consistently buy the same colors and types of clothing?

- run on autopilot and wonder why you ended up in a particular place or doing something you didn't intend to?

- rely on tried-and-trusted routines rather than explore new ones?

- stick to familiar comforts rather than challenge yourself?

While our mind is busy creating thoughts, feelings, attitudes, beliefs, and memories, the brain plays a central role in translating them into electrical and chemical signals that send complex communications to the rest of the body using hormones and neurotransmitters. It also consolidates and stores the memories of all our experiences. In addition to these roles, the brain's main functions are to maintain balance within the body, be vigilant for external cues, be efficient, and above all keep us safe from danger. The brain is very busy!

Much of the time the brain can act automatically, which makes our lives easier and more efficient. It can memorize functions and habits, such as getting up in the morning and automatically reaching for a toothbrush and toothpaste or driving a car, allowing the conscious mind to be "offline" to focus on other things. However, our brain is hypersensitive to danger signals and perceives any disruption to its regular functioning as various degrees of stress. It is our mind that gives meaning to a situation after perceiving external cues and decides whether we react in fear or in trust. When we interpret a situation as dangerous, our brain turns on the fight-or-flight reaction instantly. Built-in protective mechanisms—such as an increase in blood pressure, heart rate, and blood sugar levels—allow us to react quickly to danger or threat. In this way, short-term stress keeps us out of harm's way and protects us.

This high level of vigilance has been beneficial to humans as we've evolved, allowing us to survive actual threats such as attacks from predators, infections, and countless natural disasters. However, while our frontal brains have become larger and more sophisticated over time—leading us to explore space, develop medical robotic surgery, and create advanced computer technology—the primitive brain responsible for our fear reaction has remained basic in design. While most of us no longer have to worry about being the next meal for predators in the jungle, our mind often creates thoughts of guilt, anger, fear, resentment, and being "busy" that can create the same fear reaction provoked by the sight of a saber-toothed tiger. Our mind's automatic thoughts, or remembered sounds, sights, or smells of danger, can turn on the fight-or-flight reaction. In other words, the mind creates stress and the brain activates our body's stress hormones. By thought alone, the brain can be tricked into sending visceral messages to the body about a threat that is not actually present.

Sometimes the memory of danger can become so embedded in the brain after many repetitions that it becomes automatic, such that we continually react to a perceived instead of an actual threat. Perpetual thoughts of stress, whether real or imagined, keep our stress hormones continuously activated. And prolonged, chronic stress shrinks the brain and causes a profound change in its chemistry, biology, and electrical circuits—changes that affect our memory, mood, and functioning. To understand why, we need to know a bit about our brain.

BRAIN FUNCTION AND ANATOMY 101

The central nervous system (CNS) is the control center for the whole body and comprises the brain and spinal cord (Figure 2.1). The nerves are bundles of fibers and receptors that sense changes within our body (for example, a feeling of hunger) and our external environment (for example, the sound of screeching tires). The nerves send these messages to the CNS to be interpreted. Nerves outside our brain and spinal cord make up the peripheral nervous system, a complex information highway that comprises the somatic nervous system and the autonomic nervous system (ANS).

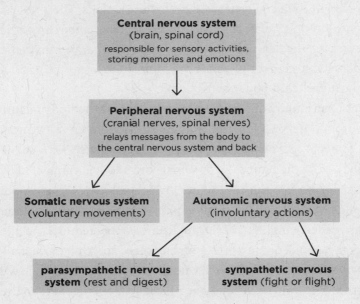

Figure 2.1. The central nervous system and its branches

Our Voluntary and Involuntary Brain:
The Somatic and Autonomic Nervous Systems

The somatic nervous system sends messages from our central nervous system to our organs, muscles, and skin when we decide to do something. It controls our *voluntary* movement. For example, we use it every time we take a big bite out of a juicy hamburger. Our somatic nervous system sends the message from our brain to our body to pick up and bite into that burger. The somatic nervous system directs the nerves that coordinate this action. These are all choices we make; they are voluntary responses rather than automatic reactions.

But what starts our mouth watering when the food arrives? What stimulated our hunger in the first place? What gets our heart pumping when we jog? These functions are under the control of the ANS, which controls our *involuntary*, or automatic, reactions. We don't always choose these actions. The ANS has two arms to regulate the involuntary functions in the body—the sympathetic nervous system (SNS) and the parasympathetic nervous system (PNS)—and their interaction forms the basis of the mind-brain-body connection.

Communication between the brain and the body occurs through nerve pathways, and an autonomic nerve pathway connects two nerve cells (neurons) (Figure 2.2). One cell is located in the brainstem or spinal cord and it is connected by nerve fibers to the second cell, which is located in a cluster of nerve cells called an autonomic ganglion (more than one are called ganglia). These ganglia are connected to a specific organ, gland, or muscle by a further set of nerve fibers. Signals travel from one cell to another along the nerve fibers, often down from the brain to the body and back up from the body to the brain.

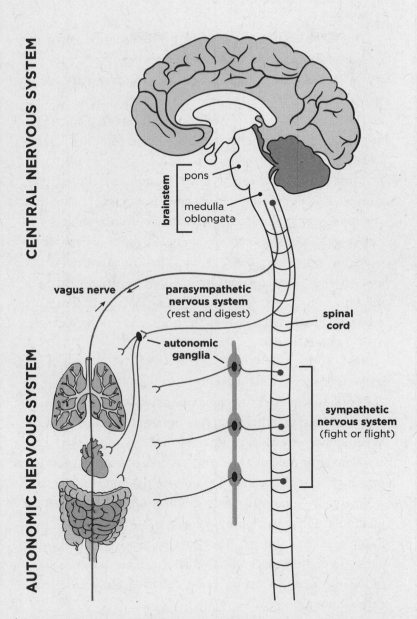

CENTRAL NERVOUS SYSTEM

brainstem

pons

medulla
oblongata

vagus nerve

parasympathetic
nervous system
(rest and digest)

spinal
cord

autonomic
ganglia

AUTONOMIC NERVOUS SYSTEM

sympathetic
nervous system
(fight or flight)

Figure 2.2. The connection between the autonomic nervous
system and the brain

One of the main nerve pathways that connects the ANS to the body is the vagus nerve, which is also known as the "wandering nerve" because this long nerve has the widest distribution in the body. It travels from the brain into organs in the neck, chest, and abdomen. The tenth of twelve cranial nerves (meaning they originate in the brainstem), the vagus nerves come in a pair but we refer to them in the singular form.

Most of the time, the ANS works automatically, without conscious thought. It determines how fast our heart beats, how vigorously our stomach contracts, and how much air gets into our lungs. It also responds automatically to our subconscious thoughts, which communicate with the ANS at every instant, and determines whether our stress hormones are turned on or off. Although the ANS is an automatic system for the most part, our mind has dominance over the brain and can regulate the ANS to a great degree.

➤ Homeostasis: Balancing the Gas with the Brakes
I often like to compare the autonomic nervous system with a car engine. The sympathetic nervous system functions to stimulate—or rev up—the body, so I refer to it in this book as "the gas." Also known as the fight-or-flight reaction, it is one of our most primitive systems, designed to prepare the body for stressful or emergency situations. The SNS allowed us to run away from predators, and these lightning-speed stress reflexes still keep us out of harm's way—such as swerving to avoid an oncoming car—on a daily basis. Our body is designed to handle this short-term stress reaction and then return to a normal, resting state called homeostasis.

When the body senses danger, the SNS is activated and the brain sends a signal to the adrenal glands to release the stress hormones adrenaline and cortisol. Activating the SNS increases heart rate, makes the heart contract with more force, and widens the airways to make breathing easier. It releases stored energy to increase muscle strength and blood sugar, and it causes the pupils to dilate. At the same time, it slows down body processes such as digestion and urination that are less important in dealing with an imminent threat.

The human body is not designed to remain revved up for long periods of time. In fact, all living things tend toward homeostasis, or equilibrium, and our bodies are no different. When our systems remain within certain pre-set limits—a body temperature of 98.6°F or a heart rate of 60 to 100 beats per minute, for example—they are better able to function optimally, which means better health. Our ancestors may have triggered their SNS regularly, but these episodes of cortisol and adrenaline surging through their bodies were mostly short-lived. Once our ancestors got away from danger, their brains deemed the external environment safe again and their heart rate slowed, their breathing eased, and their stress levels dropped. In other words, our ancestors found time to recover and soothe themselves by eating and sleeping. Most animals still do this: ducks ruffle their feathers and cats lick themselves to return to balance.

In humans, the parasympathetic nervous system (PNS) functions to inhibit—or slow down—the body and bring about this equilibrium, which is why I refer to it in this book as "the brakes." Also known as the rest-and-digest response, it releases hormones and chemicals that relax the body and allow it to recover its normal functioning. When the body is no longer under threat, the PNS is activated and the brain signals the body to release dehydroepiandrosterone (DHEA), a hormone associated with longevity and health; our happy hormone, serotonin;

and our natural painkillers, the endorphins. Activating the PNS enhances blood flow to the gut, increases contractions of the gut and release of gastric juices, and turns on secretions that aid the digestion process. At the same time, it slows our heart rate to a resting state and reduces our blood pressure by allowing our blood vessels to return to their usual diameter. In essence, almost every one of our body systems returns to a resting state. It's like putting up our feet and sipping lemonade on our porch swing.

This intricate system of gas (SNS) and brakes (PNS) operates as a series of checks and balances, ensuring that neither system dominates and that our body returns to homeostasis. In some people, this system becomes overactive (the gas is on all the time). In many of us, the ANS becomes dysfunctional and goes into alarm phase even when there's only minimal stress. Too much gas for too long will create discomfort and disease. So to address the root cause of stress-induced discomfort and disease, we must look at how our mind interacts with the ANS at every instant—how it hits the gas or pumps the brakes, depending on our internal thoughts—and learn to regulate it with conscious effort.

Understanding Stress Hormones and the Brain

Everyone has a different definition of stress, but at a basic level it refers to a state of mental or emotional strain caused by a physical, chemical, or emotional factor. Stress comes in all shapes, sizes, and quantities, and each of us perceives it differently. All of us experience daily stress, and our bodies can adapt to handle not only everyday stress but unpredictable and acute stress exposure too. For example, we encounter stress when avoiding immediate dangers such as an oncoming car—our SNS is activated, we go into a fight-or-flight reaction, and after the few seconds of fear, we realize the collision has been averted. Our PNS then kicks in, and our rest-and-digest response allows our body to relax. Some stress can even be positive: we may feel an excited adrenaline rush when skiing down a mountain, running a race, or meeting a deadline. Those events, however, are not usually sustained. When stress becomes prolonged, chronic, and excessive, it causes disease in our body. But how and why does it get that way?

➤ Our Intel Processor: The Hypothalamus

The brain has a built-in "Intel processor" called the hypothalamus, an almond-sized area at the base of the brain. Like a busy traffic cop, it is continuously scanning the environment for signs of danger, processing the information at lightning speed, and directing a multitude of functions to keep us safe. It gets us up in the morning and starts the adrenaline flowing. It controls the molecules that allow us to experience emotions such as exhilaration, happiness, anger, or upset. The hypothalamus is also a bit like a thermostat, always aiming for homeostasis. It controls how much we eat, regulates our body temperature, and acts as our "emotion detector."

The hypothalamus sends instructions to the body in two ways. First, it controls blood pressure, heart rate, breathing, digestion, and all the sympathetic and parasympathetic functions through the ANS, which speeds up or slows down body functions. Second, it regulates growth and metabolism as well as emotion by communicating with the pituitary gland, the pea-sized endocrine gland at the bottom of the hypothalamus that we often refer to as the "master gland." The instant processing mechanism of the hypothalamus works efficiently using all the senses and memory storage, which communicate with each other. Then it directs the pituitary gland to regulate our response to our environment through hormones and other chemicals. Together, they decide when to release each hormone and how much to release.

The hypothalamus and the pituitary gland also form part of the limbic system, an area of the brain that interprets emotional responses, stores memories, and regulates hormones.[1] Two key structures of the limbic system are the almond-shaped amygdala and the tiny nub called the hippocampus that lies adjacent to it. The amygdalae (there is one on each side of the brain) determine which memories are stored and where in the brain each of those memories is to be kept, and the hippocampi (there is also one of these on each side of the brain) send the memories to their assigned part of the brain for long-term storage and retrieve them when necessary.

➤ The Hypothalamic-Pituitary-Adrenal Axis

Our brain is busy and promotes efficiency. Therefore, when it comes to stress, the brain consolidates, simplifies, and anticipates any remote memory of fear or threat. The primary system for regulating the effects of stress on the body is the hypothalamic-pituitary-adrenal (HPA) axis (Figure 2.3). When the limbic system sends a message of fear or threat to the hypothalamus, it releases a hormone called corticotropin-releasing factor (CRF) in reaction to the stress. This CRF stimulates the pituitary gland, which then releases adrenocorticotropic hormone (ACTH), and in turn ACTH stimulates the adrenal glands to release cortisol.

Cortisol is just one of the hormones produced by the adrenal glands. These triangular glands, which sit atop the kidneys, have two parts: an outer part called the adrenal cortex and an

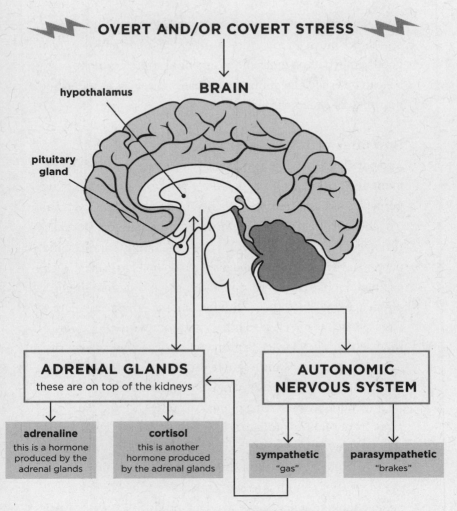

OVERT AND/OR STRESS

BRAIN

hypothalamus

pituitary gland

ADRENAL GLANDS
these are on top of the kidneys

AUTONOMIC NERVOUS SYSTEM

adrenaline
this is a hormone produced by the adrenal glands

cortisol
this is another hormone produced by the adrenal glands

sympathetic
"gas"

parasympathetic
"brakes"

Figure 2.3. How the brain communicates stress to the body

inner part called the adrenal medulla. The outer part produces hormones that are essential to life; for example, cortisol, which regulates metabolism and helps your body achieve homeostasis, as well as aldosterone, which helps to regulate blood pressure. The inner part of the gland produces the body's nonessential hormones, including adrenaline, which helps the body adapt to stress. Too much (or too little) of any of these hormones is not a good thing, but too much of the essential stress hormone cortisol can be especially damaging, because it causes a cascade of detrimental effects throughout the body.

How Stress Affects Our Health

As a physician, I realize that quantifying stress is extremely difficult and requires a lot of detective work because each of us perceives stress differently. We need to look at both external (psychosocial factors) and internal (inner dialogue, unrealistic expectations, and mindset) stressors. Simply stated, some people have *overt* stress, which seems obvious to others, such as financial hardship, broken relationships, a demanding job, physical pain, or struggles with loneliness. Others have *covert* stress, which is not clear to others and sometimes not clear to themselves. They have a healthy marriage, financial security, a wonderful house, and regular vacations, yet they develop unseen stress ulcers or drop dead of a heart attack.

Put another way, during prehistoric times, we regularly ran away from real-life predators like saber-toothed tigers (overt stress). Now we keep trying to run away from "internal" tigers, such as fears of rejection, loneliness, abandonment, and failure that roam our minds (covert stress). Negative thoughts and beliefs, including an illness mindset, produce a covert stress reaction in the body that has the same effect as overt stressors. So be very aware of the thoughts you think and the beliefs that run your program because they contribute greatly to your health. There could be a covert operation sabotaging your health!

We also need to look at people's adaptive techniques or soothing behaviors to neutralize stress and understand how they were formed. Our brains are wired for social interaction; for example, newborns learn that to acquire food they must communicate and interact with people around them. They may learn that crying results in food, whereas soft cooing is a way to obtain hugging and caressing. This early conditioning primes how our brain forms the neural circuits, or thought patterns, that process information about the world and our surroundings. When love, connection, and safety are missing, human brains perceive this as a threat, which forms a neural pathway very early in development.

Emotional threats activate the gas, yet we are mostly unaware that our subconscious thoughts are producing stress hormones even without an apparent external stressor. Having mostly adverse childhood experiences sets up neural pathways for a negative inner dialogue and a lack of soothing behaviors. For example, infants can sense when there is a lack of affection, bonding, and nurturing, which can set them up to feel neglected as adults. And children who experience verbal or physical abuse and trauma are at higher risk for disease in their later years. Their neural wiring is being set early on for anxiety, worry, and a "reactive" nervous system. In contrast, infants who are held and caressed and feel love with human touch thrive better. That relationship stability in the early years helps create a sense of security and belonging that develops neural networks that are more conducive to health and fostering better relationships.

We know that stress can show up in different forms—emotional, physical, environmental toxins, infections—but the bottom line is that an endless supply of stress hormones, no matter what their source, damages our body. When we experience chronic stress, the ANS gets stuck in the gas mode and it's like having your "pedal to the metal." Our body was not meant to be in a perpetual stress cycle without time for recovery. Cortisol and adrenaline surge through our blood vessels, and they affect almost every tissue in the body including the brain (ironically, the same organ that triggered their production). Why? The neural pathway carrying information from the ANS overlaps with the neural pathway carrying specific memories with associated emotions from the limbic system. In other words, the brain cannot discern between *real* physical or emotional threats and *perceived* emotional ones. When excessive amounts of the chemicals that mobilize the body for an emergency circulate in the body for too long, they reinforce memories with extra strength so the body never forgets them. In effect, the stress hormones cause many changes in the brain. The neural pathway gets hijacked, and subconscious memories can cause a flood of stress hormones even when we are relaxing.

While the prefrontal cortex of our brain has become highly sophisticated, the brainstem, where many of the ANS pathways begin, has not evolved at the same pace and remains primitive. It does not discern the difference between physical threats and thoughts of anger or jealousy. It processes all these negative emotions as danger signals.

Our brain has a more negative bias than a positive one. While some animals that have escaped a near-fatal attack can literally ruffle their feathers and move on, human brains can re-create a stressful event by thought alone. Stress pathways become hardwired. We look for what is missing. We focus on the worst-case scenarios and worry about outcomes that have not happened yet. We forecast the future rather than live in the present. Worse than that, we have a rewind button that automatically replays old tapes of bad memories. This potent combination leads to ongoing surges of stress hormones. Chronic exposure to stress hormones affects the brain, both directly and indirectly.

➤ Direct Effects of Chronic Stress on the Brain

The nervous system uses a system of nerve cells, or neurons, to take up, process, and transmit information through electrical and chemical signals (Figure 2.4). The brain alone contains about 100 million neurons and 100 trillion connections.[2] Each of these cells, which is about a tenth the diameter of a human hair, has three parts. The dendrites are treelike branches that receive input from other neurons. The cell body is attached to the dendrites and contains the DNA of the cell. The axons are wires of various lengths that carry electrical impulses at high speeds toward dendrites of other neurons. These impulses—which carry either excitatory (encourages neurons to fire) or inhibitory (discourages neurons from firing) messages—are transmitted across a gap called a synapse.

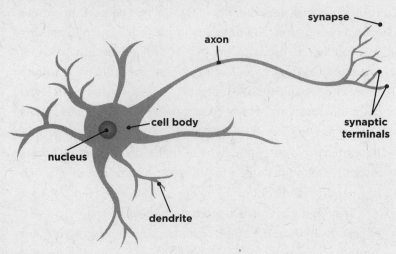

Figure 2.4. Anatomy of a neuron

Science reveals that neurons that "fire together" in a repeated pattern establish permanent neural pathways: they "wire together." The communication between neurons is carried out by a number of neurotransmitters. Some cause arousal in the brain, others drowsiness; some focus your attention, others are associated with memory and mood. Over time, exposure to chronic levels of stress hormones changes our neural chemistry and the size and shape of parts of the brain.

Chronic stress changes our neural chemistry by altering neurotransmitters such as serotonin and dopamine. Ordinarily, serotonin is an inhibitory neurotransmitter that stabilizes our mood and balances the number of excitatory neurotransmitters being fired into our brain. Dopamine is usually the "feel-good" chemical that can be both an inhibitory and excitatory neurotransmitter. If our dopamine levels are balanced, our body can reduce any symptoms of anxiety, depression, and stress. But when we are anxious and under chronic stress, the brain begins to produce an overabundance of fear-related neurotransmitters, such as adrenaline and norepinephrine, and fewer neurotransmitters associated with happiness and relaxation, such as dopamine and serotonin. To compensate, the brain creates more receptors to handle the extra fear neurotransmitters and fewer serotonin receptors, which it deems less necessary. The result is that we feel anxious more often than we feel relaxed. Some people can live in a perpetual fight-or-flight reaction, while others have such extreme anxiety they develop a panic disorder, which may require medication.

Chronic stress can also directly change the shape and size of certain areas in the brain. In neuroscience, we call this ability of the brain to change in shape and size *neuroplasticity*, and it can be both positive and negative. Long-term exposure to the stress hormone cortisol appears to cause brain neurons to shrink and interferes with their ability to send and receive information. As a result, the hippocampus becomes smaller—stress actually shrinks our brain! On the one hand, stress affects our ability to retrieve information, pay attention, or stay focused. On the other hand, the amygdala, the center for the fear reaction, becomes enlarged in chronically stressed people. We become more anxious and more fearful, and those neurons then start to wire together. For example, using MRI scans we can see that the shape and size of various brain structures are different in individuals who have post-traumatic stress disorder (PTSD).

► Indirect Effects of Chronic Stress on the Brain

Indirectly, stress hormones cause changes in the gut (our second brain) as well as in many other systems in the body. The gut damage from stress is especially relevant to the brain for several reasons. It impacts the production of serotonin, since our gut manufactures between 80 and 85 percent of our body's serotonin. Gut damage causes local inflammation that eventually finds its way to the brain and other organs. And stress appears to interfere with the way the bacteria in our gut communicate with our brain. Stress hormones also cause lack of sleep, wearing down the normal capacity of the brain to detoxify and repair itself from daily use. Overall, chronic stress exposes the brain to more inflammation.

Another indirect effect of stress on the brain is the poor diet choices made by people under stress. Stressed individuals tend to eat poorly or snack on junk food, drink more alcohol, or even abuse drugs (both prescription and recreational), which exposes the brain to more toxins. Stressed people tend to become sedentary. Lack of regular exercise is also detrimental to the brain, since the increased blood flow during exercise is good for circulation and oxygenation.

Chronic stress also changes electrical brain waves, which we can measure with an electroencephalogram (EEG) machine. When excessive cortisol disrupts the electrical wave patterns, it changes the neurochemicals in the brain, which causes arousal or alertness. Chronic stress can disrupt our sleep-wake cycles and change our normal circadian rhythms. Sleep deprivation is common in people with unresolved stress. Chronic sleep deprivation is a health risk for heart disease and diabetes and negatively affects brain memory and concentration, leading scientists to correlate it with dementia.

Remember, however, that our mind has dominance over the brain and can regulate the ANS to a great degree. To achieve health, we must learn to pump the brakes and turn off the constant flow of gas. We can cultivate a healthy brain by being aware of our beliefs and internal thoughts. By learning to challenge automatic thoughts, we can consciously replace them with intentional ones, which creates new neural thought patterns. New thought patterns lead to different behavioral choices, which first become traits and eventually turn into habits. When these thought patterns include a health mindset and positive beliefs, they are the foundation for long-term physical and emotional health.

HOW TO SHORT-CIRCUIT STRESS HORMONES AND CREATE A HEALTHY BRAIN

To create better neural pathways, we have to voluntarily or consciously put on the brakes to help neutralize the stress response. To do this, we need to remain aware of our automatic thoughts and choices—catching them before they enter our mind and chasing them out if they sneak in. Our ability to choose one thought over another is one of the most powerful tools we have.

Tap into Your Conscious Brain

The negativity bias hardwired in our brains evolved to allow us to have an indelible memory of negative and fearful experiences, reducing the likelihood we would come to harm in the future. In other words, the brain developed systems that would focus our attention on danger so that we would respond to it. In psychologist Dr. Rick Hanson's words, our brain is like Velcro for negative experiences (that is, they stick well) and like Teflon for positive ones (that is, these memories are not as "sticky"). Research suggests we are three to five times more likely to remember negative experiences than positive ones.[3] Therefore, says Hanson, to embed the "good stuff" we have to consciously secure and store positive experiences into our memories using all our senses.[4] He calls this technique "taking in the good."

Though we naturally tend to amplify negative, traumatic memories, we can do the same for pleasant experiences. When we taste, smell, touch, and feel good experiences, we amplify those experiences and their stored memory, and we can recall those positive memories at will to help neutralize some of the traumatic events. Some people are already hardwired this way or have already consciously or subconsciously cultivated a mindset that focuses on the good stuff. Others can acquire this skill when they become aware of their thought processes. Yet others remain focused on threats and fears and go through life with a big rain cloud over their heads not realizing that their subconscious is running their life story.

➤ Turn a Negative Bias into a Positive One:
  Story, Savor, Smile

Motivational speaker Mel Robbins talks about the importance of story, savor, and smile as three ways to change the way the brain encodes a memory.[5] How do we relate the events to our subconscious? What is our story? Are we the victim? Do we feel hopeless and trapped? Can we recognize a pattern? When good things happen, our negativity bias means we are less likely to pay much attention. Yet, the mind is a powerful storyteller with a vivid imagination full of pictures and sensory information. When the mind is collaborative, it tells a positive story and remembers the event as positive for future use. Feel-good chemicals flood the body each time the story is told.

To reinforce a positive story, Robbins recommends we savor, or make a conscious effort to create and embed, those positive experiences. Research supports that idea: prolonged activation of a brain region called the ventral striatum is directly linked to sustaining positive emotions and reward.[6] For example, if you win a running race (or receive recognition), take the time to revel in the admiration, enjoy the sense of accomplishment, praise yourself for your effort, and enjoy the honor rather than minimizing the event to go on to the next goal. Enjoy and savor it on a multisensorial level: hear the cheering crowds, appreciate the weight of the medal around your neck, welcome the warmth of the sun on your back, embrace all the hugs afterward. Don't focus on the next race you will enter. If you don't stop to savor the moment, your mind will gloss over this success and your brain will not hardwire the memory.

To further enhance a memory, smile. A smile is a natural human response to something pleasant. We use muscles to smile, and we memorize the positive emotion that goes with the smile. Once you have a good story memory and you have savored it on a sensory level, use your smile muscles to further embed the memory. So even when you may not feel like smiling, the physical act of smiling triggers a more positive signal in the brain because of muscle memory. When it comes to smiling, "fake it till you make it" is not a bad thing when the alternative is a negative mindset setting you up for disease.

TRY THESE ADDITIONAL STEPS to master your conscious brain mindset.

➤ Train Your Brain
Creating a health mindset uses the principles of neuroplasticity to emphasize the relationship between learning and "brain training." Just like any muscle, we can train our brain by doing "mind reps." The key to forming new neural networks is to observe our patterns of inner dialogue and change our vocabulary from criticism and judgment to encouragement and compassion. I find it helpful to start my day by setting an intention to mindfully catch and observe my thoughts. At least eight to ten times each day, I try to become aware of my automatic pathways and consciously change my vocabulary if it is negative. For example, I might try to use the word "learning" instead of "failing." If you are struggling, you could use the phrase, "I haven't mastered a health mindset yet," inferring that with time it will happen. "Not yet" is a wonderful way to reassure the brain that we are making progress. Discerning the phrase "room for improvement" from "failure" helps our inner critic be more encouraging and compassionate.

When we practice mindful meditation, we allow the mind to go quiet. As we observe our thoughts, we gain more conscious control over what thoughts we allow. The relaxed brain becomes more receptive to new learning, because neuroplasticity is more effective when the mind and body are in rest-and-digest mode.[7] Meditation alters our neural chemistry, transforms our electrical brain waves, and enhances blood flow to areas of the brain that encode memory. All of these conditions are perfect for embedding new behaviors.

Counseling tools such as cognitive behavioral therapy (CBT), neuro-linguistic programming (NLP), emotional freedom technique (EFT), and many other reframing techniques are available to help us gain more control over our emotions. CBT is used to help people with a variety of mental health disorders overcome distorted thought patterns (cognitive) and impact their actions (behavior). NLP is a therapy that connects neurological processes, language, and behavior patterns to create change to meet specific therapeutic goals. EFT is a therapy that brings together a variety of alternative medicines, including tapping and energy, to treat both physical and psychological disorders. Tapping specific acupressure points seems to allow some patients to regain control of the disordered brain waves associated with anxiety. That is, EFT aims to understand the subconscious thoughts and beliefs that underlie our choices, so we can ensure they are beneficial to our health.

The key to all of these techniques is that by understanding how and why our negative thoughts arise, we can consciously replace them with new patterns of thinking. When we do this frequently and repetitively, the new thought patterns become automatic neural circuits that benefit our brain, our ANS, and our overall health and well-being. Although CBT is quite well established, most psychiatrists do not yet fully endorse NLP and EFT, and more data and research will be needed before they are widely used. However, their ability to address subconscious beliefs as well as conscious ones makes them interesting areas to explore, and many patients have already benefited from these techniques.

Learning is the "journey" and more important than the destination. If we emphasize learning *well* over learning *fast*, we garner better results. Reinforce the new learned behavior by using reflection techniques to embed the "good stuff" and enhance the memory. Take the time to replay positive emotions such as pride and inspiration and to re-experience the situation using all your senses. The more often we choose to self-accept, self-approve, and self-appreciate, the more that behavior becomes part of our internal hard drive. Thus, we need to reward the actions we have taken, not the thoughts we passed through our brain.

➤ Neurobic Exercises

Just as we do aerobics to activate and tone our muscles, we can do brain exercises (neurobics) to stimulate our senses in new and unexpected ways.[8] Our efficient brain runs on autopilot most of the time: every day we pretty mindlessly wake up, brush our teeth, take a shower, use the same route to work. When you change up the routine, the brain has to become more conscious and aware of your mind. So neurobic exercises not only engage the conscious mind, they also help to grow new neural circuits.

In his book *Keep Your Brain Alive*, neurobiologist Dr. Lawrence Katz suggested eighty-three exercises to increase mental fitness. Each exercise met two criteria. First, it had to use one or more senses in a new way. For example, he suggested brushing your teeth with your eyes closed or with your nondominant hand. Second, it had to break a routine in an unexpected way that evoked an emotion such as happiness, love, or anger. For example, he suggested taking a new route to work or riding your bike instead of driving or taking the bus.

When you brush your teeth with your eyes closed, you rely on touch and sound rather than sight to guide your hand to the toothbrush, the toothpaste, your mouth, and your teeth. You likely pay more attention to the layout of your bathroom and the smell of the toothpaste. Neurobic exercises cause the brain's attentional and emotional circuits to become alert. They activate little-used nerve connections and keep your neural pathways active and healthy.

➤ Slow Down the Nervous System

How we form healthy brain habits is based on individual preference and a bit of trial and error. If you have great difficulty focusing or paying attention because your thoughts are too rapid or pressured, seek out a professional to help. Know that what works for some may not work for others; however, deep diaphragmatic breathing is a good place to start to slow down the nervous system and turn on the brakes.

You may already practice relaxation techniques such as meditation, deep breathing, or yoga. If so, pick one or more of them and slow your nervous system. If not, sign up for a class or ask your health practitioner, a friend, or family member for advice. Less gas and more brakes allows your brain to function better. Other ways to slow down the nervous system include sleep, which bolsters memory, mood, and concentration by detoxifying some of the by-products from brain cells and improving circulation. Exercise increases the flow of blood to the brain, bringing more oxygen and brain-derived neurotrophic factor (BDNF), which promotes the growth of neurons (brain cells).

Our brain has two hemispheres, and the two sides appear to function differently. Many of us spend a large part of our lives in "left-brain activity," which means a lot of verbal, analytical, and ordering tasks. This is our reading, writing, computing brain. For many people, engaging in "right-brain activity" is relaxing. It is visual, intuitive, and creative. Listening to music, for example, soothes the brain and can activate neural pathways and alter brain-wave patterns in ways that speech and movement cannot, bringing blood flow to areas of the brain not used in other body functions. In fact, doing any hobby you love, such as sitting in nature, painting or sculpting, or playing a musical instrument, stimulates the different centers in the brain that produce calming neurotransmitters. Indulge in regular small pleasures, do things that give you joy, set and meet goals, and above all cultivate meaningful relationships. These are all different ways to embed a program of positive calm, trust, and happiness.

Finally, sometimes just say no. Many of us get caught up doing things because people expect us to or because we are conditioned to "not disappoint" others. Sometimes saying "no" to something or someone means saying "yes" to yourself. That can be a good thing for you and your brain.

The Benefits of a Healthy Brain

The pursuit of happiness is a global desire. A happy, calm, and content brain promotes better physical health. Genetics, life events, achievements, social relationships, and even the weather contribute to how happy we are. More importantly, how our mind reacts to our circumstances and continually adjusts the default setting to trust instead of fear is the key to promoting a happy, calm, and positive brain. A brain that wakes up with a purpose beyond survival, fear, or meeting our personal needs increases life satisfaction dramatically.

A healthy brain is an essential component of a healthy body. It is the automatic computer, after all. Feeling positive seems to benefit our heart, immune system, blood pressure, and inflammatory response, just to name a few body systems. A healthy brain consolidates more memory and has better concentration, more focus, and improved creativity. A healthy brain ensures we make better automatic decisions, are quicker to respond to external cues, and are more open to growing new neural pathways. When a brain is relaxed and receiving optimal blood supply, good nutrition, and adequate sleep, it has incredible potential for growth and longevity. Healthy brains are generally happier and more adaptable.

CONCLUSION

Our brain is complex, and we often misunderstand, grossly underestimate, and sometimes oversimplify how we think it works. What we do know is that when it comes to creating health, we can harness the immense potential of the brain if we learn to use the mind as a powerful programmer. This is why it is imperative to manage chronic stress so we can engage our conscious mind to "wake up" and give the brain more effective programs to run when the old automatic ones are causing us distress. When we consciously prune bad neural circuits that get us in trouble, "upload" new programs that promote health, and add stress-management "upgrades" to the existing systems, we can use the brain's automatic, efficient, and subconscious pathways to carry out these new patterns. The goal is to make health a habit that we no longer have to "think" about because our brain simply executes it by default.

It behooves us, then, to maximize our brain's efficiency by taking care of it physically (wear a helmet; get proper sleep; avoid toxins such as through good diet), taking care of it emotionally (give it rest such as with relaxation and unplugging from technology), and using it in different ways (be creative). If you find it difficult to slow down your brain waves and optimize brain chemistry, read on. Breathing deeply while using mantras or repeating a word is an effective way to slow down and take control of your brain and your conscious mind.

3.

Mind Your Breath

Breath is the bridge which connects life to consciousness, which unites your body to your thoughts.
Thích Nhất Hạnh

SELF-ASSESSMENT

Many people use only one-third of their lung capacity. They habitually use poor breathing techniques, unaware that their shallow breathing is causing stress and that this stress is causing shallow breathing. Shallow breathing can turn into panic attacks, which cause dry mouth and fatigue, aggravate respiratory problems, and can be a precursor for cardiovascular issues.

Do you:

· feel stiff or have difficulty when trying to breathe deeply?

· have tense shoulder and chest muscles?

· feel tired or complain of dry mouth?

- have a sense of impending anxiety?

- feel breathless on exertion?

- panic or hyperventilate when anxious?

- lift your shoulders and upper chest noticeably when breathing?

- feel your breath is out of control?

- speak quickly, as all in one breath?

- have trouble finishing sentences at full volume or get breathy or lose the end of sentences?

- hold your breath to think or do something?

Our respiratory system differs from all other body systems. Organs such as the brain, heart, kidneys, and skeleton are all in good working condition while we float around in the womb before birth. The lungs do not function until we take our first breath after we're born. That first gasp of air signifies the start of a lifetime of breaths, and our last breath represents the end of our life. Breath is the essence of life itself and we breathe life into our body approximately 23,000 times a day.

Before attending the Mind/Body Medical Institute at Harvard University, I thought breath was so innate to our existence that we didn't need to learn how to do it. Yet most of us do not breathe properly. We have shallow breathing or hold our breath in our tense bodies, and we fail to connect proper breathing to health and longevity. Controlling how we breathe is one of the most important biological functions we can use to regulate our autonomic nervous system (ANS). Dysfunctional breathing can change our biology, our brain waves, our heart rate, and even our blood pressure. More importantly, poor breathing is associated with a shorter lifespan.

Every cell in our body depends on the life-giving oxygen molecules that our lungs absorb and transport through the bloodstream to our tissues. Because all organs depend on oxygen, poor oxygen supply causes major illness. So how does stress sabotage our breathing? To understand how this works, it's helpful to know a bit about the anatomy of the respiratory system.

BREATHING ANATOMY 101

Breathing, or respiration, is a system of gas exchange that supports our whole body. We breathe in oxygen from the air around us and we breathe out carbon dioxide from our body, using a respiratory system that comprises airways, sites of gas exchange, and a mechanism to induce the ventilation (Figure 3.1).

Our mouth and nose form the entry points for gas coming into the respiratory tract. These airways filter, warm, and humidify air to adapt it to the body's internal environment. Once inside the body, the air must travel into the respiratory tract, whereas food—which also enters the body through our mouth—has to be diverted from the airway and pushed into the digestive tract. The epiglottis is the guard at this crucial intersection. Though it plays an honorable role, it is only a flap of cartilage overhanging the entrance to the voice box. As we swallow, food pushes this flap of cartilage down to cover the airway and forces food to its rightful place in the stomach. Air can flow freely past as long as we aren't trying to breathe while swallowing. Sometimes air goes into the digestive system without issue; it'll only come out as a burp from the front end or take a more pungent route to the lower exit.

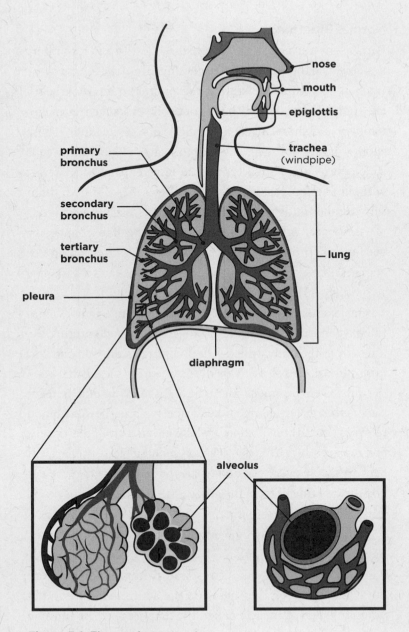

Figure 3.1. The respiratory system

Normal Breathing

Barring any mishaps, we segregate the digestive and respiratory systems, and the air we breathe continues into the lungs via the trachea, or windpipe. Picture the respiratory tract from the trachea as an inverted tree. The major trunk, or trachea, branches into two main bronchi, each leading to one of the lungs. These spongy organs are covered with a thin layer of lubricating cells called the pleura. This layer helps the lungs expand and contract without friction, just like a set of bellows. The bronchi themselves branch into many smaller bronchioles, each of which ends in a tiny air sac called an alveolus, where our cells exchange oxygen for carbon dioxide (and vice versa). A single human lung tree comprises twenty-three generations of branches and a whopping 700 million alveoli. That is a lot of gas exchange.

Gas exchange occurs in the alveoli because that's where the oxygen-rich air in our lungs meets the blood entering the lungs from the body, which is high in carbon dioxide and contains almost no oxygen. This difference in gas levels between the outside environment (air in the lungs) and our bloodstream means that gas exchange takes place: we breathe. The blood releases the carbon dioxide, a waste product from our tissues, and replaces it with oxygen. The oxygenated blood then travels back to supply every cell and tissue in the body, while the carbon dioxide travels from the lungs up through our airways and is exhaled with each breath.

Muscles do the heavy work of ventilation, which means breathing in (inhalation) and breathing out (exhalation). We don't suck in air. Instead, the respiratory muscles pull air into our chest. Between the chest and the abdomen is a thin but powerful layer of muscle called the diaphragm. The phrenic nerve originates in the neck and comes down to the chest to provide both sensory and movement signals to the diaphragm. The phrenic nerve also helps to contract other muscles of respiration such as the intercostal muscles (between the ribs). When we inhale, the diaphragm contracts and flattens, which allows the chest cavity and the lungs to expand and creates a vacuum that pulls more air into the lungs. Our chest and shoulders rise and expand, and our belly drops and pushes out. An average adult takes twelve to eighteen breaths per minute, drawing in five to eight liters of air in that time! When we exhale, the reverse happens: the muscles relax, compressing the chest, rib cage, and lungs to a smaller volume, and the pressure rises inside, forcing air out of our lungs so that just 1.2 liters remain. When we take slow, deep breaths, we engage the vagus nerve which relaxes the diaphragm and helps to turn on the brakes.

All these complex gas exchanges, muscle coordination, and air volumes must come under some central brain control. Two systems control breathing, one of which is automatic and the other of which we control (Figure 3.2).

▶ Automatic versus Conscious Breathing

The built-in automatic breathing system tells our body to breathe (try to stop breathing—it's impossible!), which is particularly useful when we are asleep or occupied with other tasks. The ANS activates this automatic impulse for breathing. Collections of interconnected neurons form "respiratory centers" in the brainstem. One such center, in the medulla oblongata and the pons, sends waves of electrical impulses that travel along the vagus nerve to the diaphragm to make it continuously contract and then relax to inhale and exhale. In turn, the vagus nerve has many nerve branches that communicate with the brain to let it know when the diaphragm is relaxed or contracted, so the brain can adjust its directions accordingly.

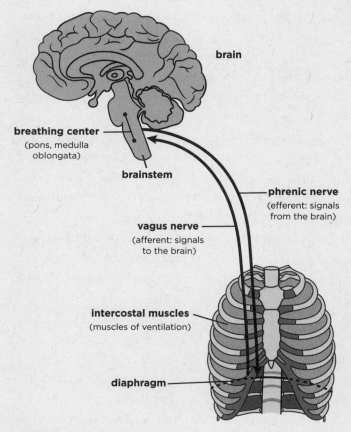

Figure 3.2. The nerve pathways for automatic and voluntary breathing

The respiratory center knows how to control the depth and rate of breathing by the amount of carbon dioxide and oxygen in the blood. For example, when you exercise, carbon dioxide levels increase and chemical receptors in the heart and throughout the arteries notify the brain to speed up the rate and depth of breathing to get more oxygen in and more carbon dioxide out. When you stop exercising, your breathing will slow and become shallower until your carbon dioxide levels return to normal. This system is known as the metabolic control of breathing.

Other respiratory centers do interesting things we might never imagine. In 2016, *Nature* published a paper that identified the cluster of neurons responsible for sighing.[1] The researchers describe a sigh as an involuntary deep breath with a remarkable purpose. The alveoli within the lungs are very fragile and prone to collapsing into their balloon-like sacs. As the alveoli deflate, our lungs lose the capacity to function. A sigh brings in air to inflate these alveoli—a necessary task the researchers say happens once every five minutes. Without the respiratory center inducing a heavy sigh, our lungs would slowly fail.

Not all respiratory functions are automatic. When we start to think about breathing, the control suddenly jumps to our conscious mind—as it likely has for you while reading about it. The impulse for voluntary breathing originates in the cerebral cortex of the brain. When we use our mind to control our breathing by deep, slow, deliberate breaths, we control the constant chatter of thoughts and regain conscious control of our inner dialogue. This ability to connect with our consciousness allows us to override the automatic circuits that are set up in the brain for breathing. We can then voluntarily breathe fast or slow, or deep or shallow, on command. However, no matter how hard we try, we cannot *stop* breathing voluntarily for more than a few minutes. Some competitive free divers, whose sport depends entirely on being able to hold their breath for long periods of time underwater, can hold their breath for nine to eleven minutes. The average for healthy humans is two to four minutes. Voluntary breathing can be overridden by involuntary respiration when the ANS or the limbic system is activated, such as when you sense danger or are triggered emotionally and the body initiates a fight-or-flight reaction.

UNDERSTANDING STRESS HORMONES AND ABNORMAL BREATHING

Many of us have lost the art of instinctual breathing. Instead, as shallow breathers, we take in less air by breathing through our mouth and holding our breath. Shallow breathing creates stress, which creates a habit of maintaining a stress posture for the muscles that support our lungs and locks us into patterns of muscle memory. We eventually forget how to breathe properly.

Dysfunctional breathing occurs for many reasons, but one of the most common is stress. When we are under stress, the fight-or-flight reaction can kick our lungs into action within seconds. This increases the diameter of our bronchi and bronchioles, maximizing the amount of airflow in our lungs. Adrenaline mediates this process and allows the lungs to bring in the most oxygen while removing carbon dioxide. The rate of breathing increases. The sympathetic nervous system (SNS) will do this whether we have had a car accident, have run a marathon, or are about to give a presentation.

Furthermore, there is a very strong relationship between breath and emotions. When we hold on to anger, grief, and anxiety it manifests in a tense diaphragm. When we hold on to physical or emotional pain, it affects our breath. Any pain turns on the SNS, because our ANS does not distinguish the kind of pain—physical or emotional. It simply reacts.

Reactions are typically poorly thought out, quick, reflexive actions driven by subconscious beliefs, biases, and judgments that are often fear-based. They are generally a protective and instinctual part of our emotional defense system, and they are accompanied by a burst of adrenaline and cortisol that increases our heart rate, respiration rate, and even blood pressure. In contrast, *responses* are calm, reasoned actions based on information gathered from both the subconscious and the conscious mind. They also take into consideration the well-being of others. Responses are accompanied by the production of oxytocin, serotonin, and gamma-aminobutyric acid (GABA), which relax us, slow down breathing, and improve circulation.

Physical and emotional pain (anxiety) trigger the fight-or-flight reaction or switch on the gas, releasing cortisol and adrenaline. These hormones rev up the body by increasing heart rate, blood pressure, and breathing. Next time you have an automatic reaction (for example, road rage), reflect and think how you could respond (for example, a deliberate, measured breath) instead. Take a deep breath before reacting, it might save you a lot of trouble!

How Stress Affects Our Breathing

➤ Asthma

Asthma, which the Greeks and Egyptians characterized as a recurrent wheeze, is a prime example of how stress affects the respiratory system. Although we do not believe stress causes asthma, we know it can trigger an asthma attack in which the airways within the lungs become altered and disrupt airflow. Both inflammation and the constant contracting of muscles within the bronchial walls temporarily block the bronchi and bronchioles. This narrowing induces the symptoms of wheezing, coughing, and shortness of breath.

We do not know the exact root cause of asthma. If you develop it before the age of twelve, it is likely genetic, whereas environmental allergens, pollution, and smoking may lead to asthma in older people. One of the most common forms is allergic asthma, which occurs when individuals with extra-sensitive airways react to allergens (pollen, dog hair, etc.) in the air. The body interprets a nonharmful substance (the allergen) as a threat and mounts an immune reaction, which means that specialized immune cells produce antibodies against the allergen. The next time the body encounters that allergen, it activates its defenses by recruiting fighter cells to the area and causing swelling and mucus within the walls of the bronchi—closing all the airways within them.

While a variety of triggers such as allergens or even exercise can bring about symptoms of asthma or even an acute life-threatening attack, stress can be a major precursor. I've seen teens entering exam season increase their use of asthma medications leading up to their finals and sharply decrease it right after the exams are over. However, we know that the SNS dilates the airways when the fight-or-flight reaction is activated, maximizing airflow to the alveoli. So, shouldn't stressful situations cause the airways to open and stop the asthma symptoms? Unfortunately, the logical conclusions about stress are inconsistent with what we see in practice—stressed-out patients have far more severe asthma.

Current thinking suggests that chronic stress causes the reacting cells in asthma to change. When they are exposed to high levels of cortisol and adrenaline, such as in a revved-up SNS system, the rational cells stop producing receptors for these stress-signaling hormones. Imagine that speakers are cranked to full blast shouting "STRESS" at each of these cells; just like a person would put in earplugs and try to ignore the racket, the cells do the same and become overwhelmed. Instead of improving the symptoms of asthma, increasing stress triggers the body. Even worse, stress starts other behaviors that worsen the condition. Thus, while we use inhaled steroids and other drugs to open the airways, stress management is an essential component in controlling and treating asthma.

Case Study: Michelle

Michelle, the CEO of a large company, was initially diagnosed with panic attacks and was eventually told she had asthma. In the months leading up to the diagnosis, Michelle had been feeling run down. She had several stressors, including marital issues, huge financial concerns, and a toxic relationship with work employees. She experienced several episodes of wheezing and coughing that were very scary for her, and one of them ended in a visit to the emergency department. She was prescribed bronchodilators and steroid inhalers, which gave her immediate relief.

During her office follow-up with me, we noted the correlation of her many stressors and her symptoms. This knowledge helped her to reframe her reaction to things such as the toxicity at work. She decided to respond rather than react to her colleagues. She practiced relaxation techniques, adjusted her sleep and diet habits, and gradually came off the daily inhalers.

Michelle still uses inhalers occasionally when she is unable to manage her stress. She noticed that when she was stressed, she picked up flus and colds more easily. Michelle became very serious about self-regulation and management. She took supplements to improve her immune system, fixed her gut health, and used techniques to help with deep relaxation breathing.

➤ Hyperventilation Syndrome and Panic Attacks

Hyperventilation syndrome (HVS) resembles and may accompany panic attacks, though the two are distinct and can exist independently. In HVS, too much air is going into and out of the lungs but we feel like we are not getting enough air, causing us to inhale and exhale deeply and rapidly. In fact, the amount of oxygen in the blood is normal; the need to gasp exists only in the mind. Panic attacks involve several additional symptoms, including increased heart rate and feelings of doom.

That's not to say HVS isn't dangerous. What's occurring is that the hyperventilation—moving large amounts of air into and out of our lungs—is taking away too much carbon dioxide from the blood. A certain amount of carbon dioxide is necessary to maintain several key body functions, including balancing the acid-base (pH) level of the blood, regulating blood flow, and acting on the respiratory centers of the brainstem to stimulate the act of breathing itself. HVS is harmful because when we lose too much carbon dioxide, we change the pH of the blood to be more alkaline. In severe cases, this change in acidity causes the nervous system to give symptoms of tingling and dizziness. The problem is that our natural reaction is to continue to hyperventilate—sending off more carbon dioxide.

Stress doesn't just worsen HVS, stress *is* the condition. The onset of true HVS has no underlying physical cause; it is entirely psychological. With a panic attack, a violent surge of anxiety and fear washes over you like a tidal wave. It feels like you're trapped, with walls inching forward and no escape. It feels like you're flailing, sinking, drowning into a sea of alarm and there's no rescue on the horizon. You think you're having a heart attack, losing your mind, maybe about to die. Your panicking mind takes over your body as your heart thumps through your chest and your breath catches in your throat. You tremble, you sweat, and you lose your balance. And this unrelenting tide of sensations only provokes more panic. If you've ever experienced a panic attack, you'll understand how it could naturally progress to the overbreathing of HVS.

Do these symptoms sound familiar? That's because the fight-or-flight reaction is being kicked into maximum overdrive during a panic attack. Massive amounts of adrenaline and cortisol enter the bloodstream to deal with the perceived threat. Without a physical release for all its energy, the body shudders and breaks down. We can stop this self-perpetuating problem by slowing down our breaths to just a couple per minute. Alternatively, a method popularized in the media is rebreathing with a paper bag. Breathing like this recirculates blown-off carbon dioxide back into our lungs and blood to restore normal levels.

Case Study: Sam

Sam, a university student, had an extreme anxiety attack while cramming for an exam. His parents were financing his education from Singapore and he was under tremendous pressure to perform academically. Just the thought of failing sent him into a panic attack, and the wheezing became so severe that it led him to the emergency department of the local hospital.

When he was assessed, his blood tests showed high levels of carbon dioxide. He was hyperventilating. He was given a paper bag to breathe into and he had some relief. He was also advised that his anxiety had escalated to a full-blown hyperventilation episode. He received a prescription for Ativan to help relieve anxiety.

He arrived at my clinic a few days later feeling less anxious, but he didn't like the drowsiness he was feeling from the Ativan. He was counseled extensively on the mind-body connection, given breathing techniques, and shown the association between stress hormones and hyperventilation. Over the next few weeks, he learned to regulate his ANS by breathing deeply, had no further episodes of hyperventilation syndrome, and no longer needed to take Ativan. He also had some counseling from student health services to reframe the expectations he had of himself.

➤ My Story

I didn't understand that I had been walking around holding my breath for the previous seven years until I met Dr. Herbert

Benson at Harvard University's Mind/Body Medical Institute. A cardiologist and the author of *The Relaxation Response*, Dr. Benson has made it his mission to teach people the importance of deep diaphragmatic breaths to induce health and reduce stress. I realized that many people, including myself, become habituated to a certain holding pattern of breathing after a particular trauma or chronic stress. In my case, I was holding on to the traumatic memory of the accident and reacting to chronic pain signals by tensing my diaphragm and other muscles.

Our emotional state is directly linked to the ANS and predicts how we hold our diaphragm. When there is fear or anxiety, the SNS activates the stress response. Shallow, upper-chest breathing using our shoulder muscles is typical when we need to fight-or-flight. Dr. Benson added that our rib cage and surrounding muscles become accustomed to shallow breathing and can, in fact, even change the shape of our chest. Human lungs have an enormous capacity to breathe in oxygen but we use only one-third of our vital real estate when we shallow-breathe.

Initially, when asked to inhale deeply, hold for a few seconds, and then exhale completely, I felt stiff and uncomfortable. Creating a habit of deep breathing took conscious effort and practice. It also meant addressing unprocessed emotions, such as fear and anger, which triggered old breathing habits. In my case, Dr. Benson urged me to create a different memory than the one I held. Instead of being crushed on the steering wheel and feeling suffocated, I visualized myself driving in a relaxed state enjoying music and taking in the gorgeous scenery.

With practice, I began to feel the muscles surrounding my chest "let go" and I could finally get a deep breath in. Since then I have improved my ability to breathe deeply. It has become a subconscious habit to take deep breaths throughout the day that can instantly bring me back to the present moment and help ground me for a speaking event or the next patient. Furthermore, having a daily meditation practice has been incredibly helpful for "undoing" the holding patterns of my breath muscles. Using relaxation response techniques three or four times a day has become a part of my routine, as it connects my emotional state to my body and it only takes a few minutes. In addition, deep breathing not only relaxes the diaphragm muscle but promotes relaxation of other body muscles.

HOW TO CULTIVATE A HEALTHY BREATH MINDSET

When we breathe voluntarily, consciously, our mind exerts tremendous control on the rate and quality of breathing, and this controlled breathing has a measurable effect on our mental state. In our crazy, digitally based, and escape-driven society, slow intentional breaths help our brain to focus and our body to relax. When we consciously relax the diaphragm with deep belly breaths, we trigger the parasympathetic nervous system (PNS), or the brakes, which releases the healthy, healing chemicals that help reduce inflammation. Brain waves slow down and the body becomes relaxed.

Re-set Your Autonomic Nervous System through Deep, Controlled Breath

Next time you feel yourself about to react to a situation, take a deep breath and step away. It's a great opportunity to recognize that only a breath separates you from an automatic reaction or a conscious response: our breath keeps us centered and in a calm state so we can respond rather than react. That is how quickly you can transform the ANS from gas to brakes. Dr. Benson's research on how stress affects the body, and his three-step Relaxation Response as a way to inhibit the fight-or-flight system and rev up the PNS, have played a major role in my own life and my understanding of healing.[2] In my clinical practice, his teachings form a key part of the mind-brain-body approach I bring to my patients' care.

Knowing that our state of mind regulates breath is a great way to feel empowered. Since stress thoughts come automatically, we have to voluntarily and consciously turn on the relaxation response to neutralize the effects of stress hormones. When we engage the relaxation response, the body shifts to a normal state of rest. Both heart rate and blood pressure normalize, as do digestion and blood flow to our extremities, as cortisol and adrenaline diminish in the blood. The ANS no longer senses a threat and the brakes come on.

When I returned to Vancouver after completing my course at the Mind/Body Medical Institute, I was inspired to reclaim my health. However, being trained in evidence-based medicine and used to relying on robust clinical trials, I had a healthy dose of skepticism. I needed more proof, so I spent a substantial amount of time and effort researching the mind-brain-body connection on my own. I studied a powerful technique called mindfulness-based stress reduction (MBSR) made popular by Dr. Jon Kabat-Zinn.[3] MBSR combines mindfulness meditation, body awareness, and yoga as well as reflection on patterns of thinking, feeling, and behavior to help people become more focused on the present and learn nonjudgmental acceptance. The program is now well established in many clinics and hospitals, and paired with relaxation techniques such as the Relaxation Response,

MBSR can physiologically lower heart rate, lower blood pressure, and improve circulation.

➤ The Breath, Mind, Word Method

My deep, controlled breathing technique combines the Relaxation Response (deep diaphragmatic breathing, progressive muscle relaxation, and repetition of a word) that I learned from Dr. Benson at Harvard and my own research on mindfulness-based stress reduction. It's a technique I've applied successfully for myself and my patients. In fact, it was this meditation and *not* medication that transformed my life after the accident and has helped me to transform the lives of thousands of my patients. Here are the three parts of my breath, mind, and word (BMW) meditation. Find a comfortable spot and sit quietly for a few minutes before you begin.

1. *Breath.* Start by inhaling slowly and deeply through the nose, holding the breath for five seconds, and then exhaling even more slowly through the mouth. Repeat these deep, slow breaths, focusing on making the exhale longer than the inhale. This deep breathing relaxes the large diaphragm muscle that separates our chest and abdomen and engages the vagus nerve to slow down the ANS.

   After breathing slowly for about two minutes, contract each muscle of the body and then slowly relax it, starting at the head and working down to the toes. Just let the body be loose and stay in this relaxed state. Science shows that a tense diaphragm and tense body muscles keep the ANS in fight-or-flight mode. When tense muscles finally relax, the brain releases opioid-like chemicals. Dr. Benson called this muscle-brain response "remembered wellness." Keep repeating these long, slow breaths before going on to the next step.

2. *Mind.* Try to become aware of the thoughts going through your mind. Often there are hundreds of automatic thoughts, many of them repeated from the day before and the day before that. Keep bringing your attention back to your breath. If you feel pain or find your thoughts automatically turning to stressors (past or future), be aware of them but just observe them. When your thoughts wander, gently bring your focus back to the breath. This reconnects the mind and body to integrate the systems and stay in the present moment. When the mind is focused on the "now," the fight-or-flight reaction turns off and your breathing becomes deeper and more controlled.

3. *Word.* Pick a soothing word (peace, amen, om) and shift your attention from your breath to silently repeating this single word as you exhale. Repeat this word until the brain becomes calm. It's sometimes said that wherever your attention flows, energy goes. Focusing your mental attention on breath and word forces the brain to change its energy. We can actually observe brain-wave patterns change from erratic, high-amplitude waves to gentle "alpha" waves.

Put these three steps together. Simply inhale, hold for five seconds, and repeat your word silently as you exhale. Keep your mind focused on the breath and the soothing word. Do this meditation for ten to twelve minutes every morning, and repeat it in the evening or throughout the day, if you find it helpful.

In this relaxed state, the brain releases endorphins (natural painkillers), melatonin (a natural sleeping pill), and serotonin (a natural antidepressant), just to name a few natural feel-good chemicals. This is the "sweet spot" when the ANS shifts from the gas to the brakes. Some people feel relaxed, calm contentment and some even feel euphoria. With frequency and repetition, the ANS is ultimately *re-set* to produce healing and repair chemicals for the body.

Know that there is no such thing as a bad meditation. Every time you try controlled breathing and focused thought, your brain gets closer to making it an automatic habit: you will get better and better at it. Just stay focused on the road and stay in your BMW!

$$\longleftrightarrow$$

TRY THESE ADDITIONAL STEPS to master your deep, controlled breath mindset.

➤ Controlled Breathing

Some people find it difficult to breathe deeply and engage their mind at the same time, as BMW requires. That's okay. Focus only on the breath. When we pay attention to our breath, it forces us to be in the present moment. This forces us to be mindful and conscious so we stay in control. Still not convinced? Navy Seals learn controlled breathing techniques during training. It helps them to focus and remain calm and nonreactive in high-stress situations. Across the country, police forces teach their officers controlled breathing techniques to deal with the trauma they witness. If these individuals, who encounter extreme situations of stress including life and death, have learned to use breath as a significant coping tool, perhaps we can learn from them. And practice makes perfect when it comes to intentional breathing and learning to turn on your PNS. If at first you don't succeed, try, try again!

➤ Use Guided Breathing Exercises

If you're new to controlled breathing or even if you're not, some people find it helpful to follow guided exercises. Some great apps for your phone are Headspace, Calm, and Breathe. Headspace is useful to learn meditation and practice breathing and relaxation techniques. It can be used three to four times per day for one- to two-minute mini-meditations to re-set the ANS. Calm is very popular for relaxation, meditations, and improving sleep and mood. Some people say it helps them to get out of left-brain thinking and into their right brain, where they feel more creative. Breathe is a particularly good way to remind you to take deep breaths periodically throughout the day. It offers a focal point to help achieve steady control over a rapidly changing environment and a reactive ANS.

Muse is a wearable headband fitted with sensors that measure the brain's electrical signals. The app that comes with the device converts the brain's electrical signals into audio that you hear through headphones. If your mind tends to wander off, Muse helps you to regain your focus within milliseconds. The headband helps you reach a deeper state of relaxation because the various sounds it plays train your brain to stay in a meditative state rather than in "busy brain" state.

The Benefits of Controlled Breathing

Almost every relaxation technique involves controlling the breath, whether it is yoga, meditation, or stretching. When we learn to breathe properly and hold the diaphragm in the proper position, this helps to regulate stress hormones through a feedback system to the ANS. This controls how much disruption occurs to the body's immune system, cardiovascular function, and gut, just to name a few of the systems affected by stress. Learning to breathe properly also improves our longevity because of the improved oxygenation and the healing hormones it produces in contrast to shallow breathing. Proper breathing can also bring about healing to any pre-existing condition in the body.

Scientists at Stanford University identified a special cluster of neurons in the brainstem that connect breathing to different states of mind.[4] This research provides some understanding of how breath quality, rate, and depth are connected to our emotions, because it suggests a link between respiration and "pacemaker" neurons in the brainstem. Research is still pending on whether yawning, gasping, laughing, sobbing, sighing, excitable breathing, or slow, relaxed breathing are each associated with a different cluster of neurons. However, deeper understanding may give us very precise means of treating disordered breathing and emotional states in the future, with possible therapies for stress, depression, or automatic negative thoughts.

Dr. Benson's research provides some clues. For example, in a control group that was practicing his Relaxation Response, 50 percent of the subjects were subsequently able to reduce their blood pressure medication. His studies also concluded that women who regularly practiced the relaxation response several times a day reported less anxiety, better mood and sleep, and even fewer, less-intense hot flashes. The most compelling findings were that the relaxation response elicited chemicals that reduced inflammatory markers and altered the messages in certain genes, such as those of patients with type 2 diabetes.[5]

In other words, Dr. Benson's work reinforced the idea that our psychology profoundly affects our biology at every level. Furthermore, he noted that slower, deeper breathing lowers blood pressure, improves gut function, and even improves EEG recordings, proving to the medical community that we can regulate the ANS. He showed that turning up the PNS (brakes) can counteract the detrimental SNS (gas) by producing a different chemical outcome in the body. The hormones of stress are neutralized with deep breathing. We produce more serotonin, endorphins, and GABA in the brain.

Deep, controlled breathing techniques have many benefits that include

· a better ratio of oxygen and carbon dioxide in the blood,

· slower heart rate and lower blood pressure readings,

· reduced levels of cortisol and adrenaline in the blood,

· improved physical energy,

· better oxygenation of body tissues,

· better muscle function by reducing lactic acid,

· better immune system function,

· a better emotional state, a sense of calm and well-being,

· improved digestion and gut function,

· improved aging and longevity, and

· possibly even modified gene expression, according to new research.[6]

CONCLUSION

We come into this world with a breath in and we leave this world with a breath out. Everything in between is life! Although we can't control whether or not we breathe, we can control *how* we breathe. We are born with a natural tendency for deep belly breathing, yet somehow between childhood and adulthood most of us lose this capacity. Effective exchange of oxygen from air to the bloodstream sustains every cell in our body. Therefore, while disordered breathing is often a result of stress, consistently tense respiratory muscles lead to "automatic" shallow breathing. Shallow and improper breathing decreases the amount of oxygen in our body, interrupts our sleep, limits our muscular stability and movement, and leads to ill health and disease.

A significant key to health is practicing breathing techniques that optimize respiration and gas exchange and maximize our heart and lung reserves by improving our PNS control. Deep, controlled diaphragmatic breathing—using our belly and chest muscles—is an excellent way to exert some control over our ANS and ensure all our tissues get oxygen for healing, especially the brain. When we have controlled breathing, we become present and our mind slows down so we make more conscious decisions about what we think, say, or do. In other words, if you feel agitated, anxious, unfocused, and distracted, or you simply want to improve your health . . . just breathe!

4.

Mind Your Gut

All disease begins in the gut.
Hippocrates

SELF-ASSESSMENT

The gut, which is more formally known as the digestive system or the gastrointestinal tract, is our second brain. Many of us struggle with gut-related issues and don't realize how much these issues affect our overall health and well-being. We end up with debilitating medical issues that we don't connect to the gut issues that were the first warning signs.

Do you:

· experience chronic diarrhea, constipation, gas, bloating, heartburn, or upset stomach?

· have gut-related disorders, such as irritable bowel syndrome (IBS) or inflammatory bowel disease (IBD)?

· often get colds or the flu?

· experience headaches, brain fog, or memory loss?

- experience sleep disturbances and excessive or constant fatigue?

- have skin rashes and other skin problems such as acne, eczema, or rosacea?

- crave sugar or carbohydrates?

- have arthritis or joint pain?

- undergo unintentional weight changes?

- suffer from food intolerances?

- have nutritional deficiencies?

Do you ever just get that gut feeling? That innate sense you are making the right call, or perhaps that something bad is about to happen. We have all experienced that instinctual feeling from our gut, even if we struggle to grasp why. You might circle C instead of B on an answer sheet or pass up a too-good-to-be-true offer you've been assured is "impossible to refuse." I often appreciate listening to my gut after the fact, even if I am not sure I should at the moment.

Our "thinking brain" is in our head but our "feeling brain" is in our gut. The connection is primal, and interestingly both systems originate from the same embryonic tissue before a fetus is formed. During this period when the embryo divides at a very rapid rate, a group of cells called the neural crest gives rise to the brain and spinal cord and a different section of this same tissue branches off and forms the enteric (gut) nervous system. Hundreds of millions of these neural cells line the gut, where they help the gut to contract and "sense" pressure and pain. Some sources say the nerve cells in the gut outnumber the neurons in our spinal cord and peripheral nervous system, and thus we often refer to the gut as our "second brain."[1] So the saying, "Trust your gut," really means, "Trust your second brain!" Our gut does more than intuitively sense right from wrong, however. It is integral to our physical and emotional health and deeply connected to our brain.

GUT ANATOMY 101

The gut, or gastrointestinal (GI) tract, is the intake point for all the food and fluids that our body needs to function. This tract is a continuous tube that extends from the mouth to the anus, with digestive juices and secretions from various organs helping to break apart and absorb nutrients along the way (Figure 4.1). While the diameter and function of the tract varies throughout, at no point does the gut tube break or stop before finishing its course through our body. The gut walls therefore form a barrier between what's inside the tube and everything outside it. In other words, the GI tract is a contained environment in which food from outside our bodies is broken down and stored or used for energy, and anything it can't use is eliminated outside the body. In this way, the GI tract protects the sterile internal environment of our body by keeping undigested food and waste away from our vital organs and tissues.

This digestive tube is the reason humans have been able to develop such complex body systems. The first multicellular life forms were no more than life rafts of cells huddled together as they floated through the primordial oceans. Over millions of years, some organisms developed a cavity on the side of or inside their body that allowed them to ingest nutrients and hold on to them. Having ready access to more nutrients for a longer time made it easier to survive and reproduce. Some of the simplest organisms today maintain this structure. Jellyfish, for example, never swallow food; they ingest it through a cavity with a single opening, hold on to it in the cavity until enzymes digest the nutrients, and then eject the waste through the same opening they used to ingest the food.

As organisms evolved, some developed a second gut opening that meant they could ingest food at one end, use the tube running through their body to exponentially increase digestion and absorb more nutrients, and then excrete the waste at the other end. Because this more complex system enabled the consumption and conversion of more food into energy, humans developed brains, circulatory systems, and skeletons, and other species added wings and tails. With the gut at the center of our development, it makes sense that a healthy gut translates to a healthy body.

Our anatomy is organized around the gut's main function, which is to supply energy to the body. This occurs through

· digestion, the physical and chemical breakdown of our food into micronutrients, and

· absorption, the actual uptake of the molecules into our bloodstream.

Digestion begins in the mouth, where the teeth crush and churn food into smaller particles while our enzyme-rich saliva—secreted from glands in the cheeks, under the tongue, and around the jaw—begins to break it down. Humans produce about a quart of saliva per day—that's a lot of enzyme action! Once we swallow that partially digested food into our food tube (esophagus), the muscular walls of the esophagus move it through our digestive system using a process of progressive contractions known as peristalsis. The gut tube is like a long and winding road with many glands that secrete juices to aid in digestion and breakdown. From the esophagus food enters the stomach, a bag-like, muscular organ where powerful acids and enzymes known as gastric juices further break down the food into a sludge called chyme. Sphincters at either end of the stomach prevent the chyme from exiting upward or downward before it is ready to move on.

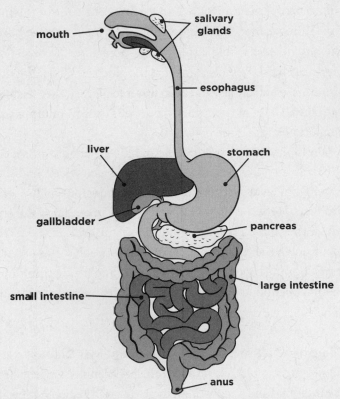

Figure 4.1. The digestive system, including the gastrointestinal (GI) tract (a.k.a. the gut)

From there, the stomach opens into the small intestine, which is about twenty feet long. This is where we absorb the most nutrients, and it takes the food several hours to pass from one end of the small intestine to the other. Along the way, secretions from the liver and gallbladder (bile) and the pancreas (digestive enzymes) help further break down the food particles into simple sugars, fatty acids, and amino acids. Small finger-like projections called villi and microvilli line the small intestine and increase the surface area of the GI tract to roughly 2,700 square feet —the area of a tennis court! The cells of the intestinal lining, called enterocytes, absorb as many nutrients from the chyme as possible, after which thousands of corresponding small blood vessels transport the glucose, lipids, minerals, vitamins, electrolytes, and even water to all the other tissues in the body. These nutrients allow our cells to grow, multiply, and support and repair the body.

From the small intestine, the remaining chyme passes into the large intestine, which is shorter but much wider. It absorbs water from what's left of the chyme, forming our body's waste products—feces. Trillions of bacteria live in our large intestine where they live off what our body doesn't use. Finally, the feces move down the tract and are expelled through the anus. At no time does the tube break, but chemical and mechanical forces modify the food so that we extract all its micronutrients and expel what we can't use.

The Gut as a Barrier and Defense against Disease

While enterocytes take up and transfer essential nutrients from the intestine and supply them to the rest of the body, they also play an important role in protecting us from disease. Picture a line of "soldier" cells standing tall and erect, shoulder to shoulder, creating a wall of tight junctions to keep the border safe (Figure 4.2). This barrier between what is inside our gut and everything outside is only one cell thick and less than one micron wide (smaller than a dust particle)!

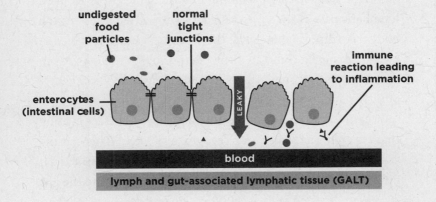

Figure 4.2. Enterocytes in a healthy gut (left) versus a leaky gut

In a healthy gut, the life-sustaining enterocytes do a fantastic job of protecting our body from toxic bacteria, chemical toxins, short-term stress, and wear and tear. Although the soldier cells are completely renewed about once a week, the key to maintaining this border security is to keep the frequency, intensity, and amount of exposure to offending agents at a minimum. These offending agents include alcohol, bacteria, viruses, toxins, and stress hormones, all of which attack the gut wall.

When the tight junctions between the enterocytes break down, these cells can no longer stand shoulder to shoulder like a line of soldiers. The physical breach in security can lead to an illness commonly called "leaky gut syndrome," in which undigested food proteins, toxins, and harmful bacteria gain access to our body. This permeability becomes a major cause of both gut problems and other inflammatory diseases in the body. Our soldiers have fallen to the enemy!

To combat breaches in the intestinal lining and other threats to our digestive system, 80 percent of the body's immune tissue lies in the gut. We call this immune capacity the gut-associated lymphatic tissue (GALT), and it plays a key role in protecting the body from disease. Much like the security systems involved in checking baggage onto an airplane, the goal of the GALT is to make certain that only "scanned" and approved materials enter our body and to expel untagged "baggage" out of the body.

Healthy human cells in the gut lining have a surface coating that our immune system can recognize as "self." This coating is known as the human leukocyte antigen (HLA) complex and it differentiates our own cells from others that come into the gut, such as undigested animal cells found in protein. Digested food, which is broken down into proteins, carbohydrates, and fats that are too small to have an immune-recognizable coating, can also pass through the GALT freely. However, infected cells, bacteria, and undigested food produce a different coating that alerts the immune system to their presence. If these potentially harmful substances make it past the enterocyte border, alarm bells will ring throughout the GALT "airport" to alert the system that an unidentified intruder is trying to make it into the body. When this happens, the GALT activates defense mechanisms to track the coating, and the immune system will tag and destroy anything that does not match the HLA complex.

Intestinal flora, or gut flora—the bacteria that inhabit our gut—work alongside the GALT. These trillions of bacterial cells outnumber our own human cells and form a vital, though often overlooked, part of our gastrointestinal system. These are not disease-causing bacteria; they help our body function better.

In fact, the normal gut microbiome—this community of micro-organisms in our gut—is helpful and influences our health, from improving immunity to improving mood.

As a newborn baby, we have a sterile gut as we emerge from our mother's womb. Within the first couple of hours and days, bacteria from the birth canal and from the surrounding environment move into their new home within our body, mainly in the gut. Maternal breast milk also contains prebiotic nutrients and probiotic bacteria that populate the infant gut, encourage the growth of "good" bacteria, and establish our personal signature microbiome, which is as unique as our fingerprints. This very important initial imprinting process "trains" the immune system so we become accustomed to these species of good bacteria and promote their growth while we simultaneously obstruct pathogenic "bad" bacteria. All these good bacteria are within us at infancy and remain present while our GALT develops further. This lymphoid tissue, which began to develop during pregnancy, eventually concentrates mostly in the small intestine but is present in pockets in most of the intestinal tissue throughout the gut.

In a healthy microbiome, the good bacteria outcompete the bad bacteria that form harmful toxins. The adult microbiome continues to produce nutrients and helps to detoxify the body by removing from the colon whatever toxic substances the liver could not clean up earlier. We often call these bacteria the "satellite liver" because the liver mainly helps to detoxify our body in addition to producing bile to break down fats in our diet. The helpful bacteria in the colon aid the body to absorb nutrients such as complex carbohydrates, calcium, and iron. They also support the production of the essential vitamin K2, which is impossible without the billions of helpful bacteria. Mucus production from the good bacteria helps us to pass stool, protect the lining, and clear waste from inside our intestines. Furthermore, the gut flora communicate with the GALT, especially when we are infants (for more on this subject, see Mind Your Immune System, Chapter 8).

The Gut as a Second Brain

The conduit for information between our gut and our brain is the vagus nerve, one of the largest of the twelve cranial nerves. It originates in the brainstem and spreads its branches to several other organs. This communication system between the brain and the gut, called the gut-brain axis, is bidirectional, meaning the signals along this pathway can originate in the gut, the brain, or both.

As it does with other systems in our body when we feel stress, the sympathetic nervous system (SNS) communicates the need to prepare our bodies for danger. In the gut, it sends the message to divert energy and blood supply from processing food (digestion) to make it available for more pressing needs such as fight or flight. Peristalsis (the speed and intensity of contractions) decreases, as does the secretion of digestive enzymes. If normal digestion is restricted frequently and for long periods of time, our body cannot properly absorb nutrients to rebuild and repair the body, supply energy, or mount a proper defense against intruders. The ultimate result is illness and inflammation.

But that's not all. One of the most rapidly evolving areas of science is neurogastroenterology, the study of the brain, the gut, and their interactions. Specifically, researchers in this field focus on the functions, malfunctions, and malformations of the sympathetic, parasympathetic, and enteric divisions of the digestive tract. In recent years, studies[2] have linked mentally altered states to inflammation in the body. Increasingly, psychiatrists have realized the profound connection between mood disorders and a sick gut. We will almost certainly see much more research on the inflammation-depression connection, as well as the influence of the gut-brain axis on chronic pain, schizophrenia, and even dementia.

Emerging research[3] has also related our gut flora and the compounds they produce to our psychiatric health. Study of the "microbiome-gut-brain axis" may lead to treatments that target changes to our microbiome to affect conditions such as depression or anxiety and to improve mood and cognitive function. For example, in the future, physicians might prescribe probiotics or supplements to restore good bacteria in the gut of patients with anxiety or depression. It is becoming clear that our microbiome has a tremendous influence that reaches far beyond the gut to affect an aspect of our biology few would have predicted—our mind!

As a pharmacist who dispensed antidepressant drugs, a doctor who prescribed them, and a patient who received them, I think there is certainly a place for drugs that help build serotonin levels in the brain to alleviate pain, anxiety, and depression. However, we must also optimize gut health since it is a crucial component of our overall well-being. Before we get too excited about eating sauerkraut to fight depression, we still need further studies to understand exactly how our microbiome contributes to the production of serotonin and how these signals are communicated to the brain.

UNDERSTANDING STRESS HORMONES AND OUR GUT DYSFUNCTION

Do you ever speak publicly to groups of people? A moment before your presentation, do you get a sudden urge to use the bathroom? This common occurrence is a perfect example of how stressful situations can affect our gut function. Just as we experience "butterflies in our stomach" or a "gut feeling" that something is wrong, this urge to use the bathroom when we are anxious is our fight-or-flight reaction acting on our gut! Short bouts of stress like this happen to everyone, and our bowels return to normal in between. However, prolonged stress without those breaks in between inflames the gut and leads to illness.

In reality, the gut nervous system can function on its own due to its trillions of nerve cells, which communicate constantly among themselves and with other parts of the gut. The brain and spinal cord also influence the gut nervous system through the sympathetic and parasympathetic nervous systems, the gas and brakes respectively, of our autonomic nervous system (ANS). Too much time on the gas burns out our engine and creates wear and tear that appears as illness and disease in the gut, initially as localized inflammation and later as systemic disease elsewhere in the body.

Inflammation literally means "fire," and while we need inflammation to protect us from infection by foreign organisms such as bacteria and viruses, this defense mechanism should not be on all the time. When inflammation occurs, chemicals from white blood cells are released into the blood or affected tissues to attack the toxins and fight off disease. This release of chemicals increases the blood flow to the area and may result in redness and warmth. Some of the chemicals cause fluid to leak into the tissues, which results in swelling. This protective process can stimulate nerves and cause pain but it protects the affected areas and allows them to ward off the attack. If inflammation persists, however, the chemicals begin to damage all the body's tissues, including the brain.

Inflammation is the universal driver of disease, both physical and mental. We now know that while stress stems from a multitude of factors including poor diet, poor lifestyle choices, external toxins, infections, heavy metals, and emotional stress, the spark of ignition for inflammation throughout the body occurs in the gut where the immune system is dominant.

How Stress Affects Our Gut Function
➤ Gastroesophageal Reflux Disease
In normal digestion, the esophageal sphincter opens to allow food to pass into the stomach and closes to prevent food and stomach juices from flowing back into the esophagus. However, chronic stress can lead to gastroesophageal reflux disease (GERD), commonly known as heartburn or acid reflux, which occurs when the sphincter weakens and stomach acid and/or stomach contents flow back up into the esophagus.

Compared with the stomach, the esophagus has a much thinner lining and lacks a protective mucous coating and therefore becomes irritated and inflamed, potentially leading to cancer or internal bleeding. Stress can increase symptoms of GERD, and the symptoms of GERD increase stress levels. The stress response blocks certain prostaglandins that are usually secreted by the stomach to protect it from acid, which causes even more discomfort.

> ➤ Peptic Ulcers

Ulcers occur when the protective layer of mucus erodes from the lining of the stomach or intestine, allowing bacteria and stomach acid to attack the bare tissue. For decades, scientists agreed that stomach ulcers resulted from stress. Then researchers Barry Marshall and Robin Warren discovered that bad bacteria called *Helicobacter pylori* were associated with stomach ulcers, and Dr. Marshall set out to prove once and for all that bacteria cause ulcers.[4] After ensuring his stomach was free from *H. pylori*, he ingested a colony of these bacteria and, sure enough, in ten days he developed gastritis, heartburn (GERD), and inflammation. This solidified his theory and the medical community accepted his argument for years. However, the Centers for Disease Control and Prevention reported that two-thirds of the population have *H. pylori* with no evidence of ulcers.[5] They concluded having *H. pylori* in your gut does not cause ulcers.

To prove whether the cause of ulcers is bacteria or stress, researchers in Denmark studied 3,300 people over several years, watching their diet, lifestyle, and stress levels.[6] Their findings were consistent with the first theory: stress is an independent predictor for ulcers. However, most of the ulcer patients also had *H. pylori*. They concluded that a constant stream of stress hormones reduces oxygen, nutrients, and mucus production in the stomach lining, allowing *H. pylori* to flourish, grow, and erode it. In other words, high levels of cortisol suppress the immune system, laying the foundation for bacteria such as *H. pylori* to dominate and lead to an ulcer.

> ➤ Dysbiosis

Dysbiosis is a condition that can occur when harmful bad bacteria outcompete and replace the beneficial good bacteria in the gut. Its symptoms include constipation, diarrhea, flatulence, and bloating, and it can result from eating a poor diet, drinking too much alcohol, repeatedly taking antibiotics, ingesting toxins or heavy metals from food, or being exposed to stress hormones for long periods of time. For example, most antibiotics kill all the bacteria in the gut, allowing harmful bacteria to recolonize a previously healthy colon. For this reason, antibiotics should be used with care, as they can be detrimental to our immune system in the long run. Dysbiosis also correlates with irritable bowel syndrome, inflammatory bowel disease, colon cancer, and even obesity.

➤ Irritable Bowel Syndrome

Irritable bowel syndrome (IBS) is a common condition that includes abdominal pain, bloating, diarrhea, and/or constipation. Although it is a debilitating illness that can last for years, IBS is not life-threatening, does not damage any of our gut walls or organs, and rarely progresses to diseases such as colon cancer. We don't know the exact causes, but there appears to be a strong association between IBS and anxiety. That is, an increase in stress levels can create physiological changes in the gut that bring on the symptoms of IBS.[7] When the stress reaction is on over a prolonged time, the blood supply from the gut is redirected to the muscles. Sometimes the fight-or-flight reaction causes overactivity in the intestinal muscle, and the rapid contractions cause diarrhea. At other times, the opposite occurs, resulting in constipation. When the fight-or-flight reaction is on constantly, it turns off the intestine's digestive functions (no time to digest when you are running from a saber-toothed tiger). Over time, the lack of gastric juices and activity in the intestinal muscle cause constipation, bloating, and abdominal pain.

The symptoms of IBS themselves (i.e., pain and diarrhea) are significant stressors. In fact, diagnosed depression and anxiety often coincide with IBS, and studies have shown that traumatic experiences during childhood, such as physical or sexual abuse, can increase our risk for developing IBS in adulthood.[8] Some evidence suggests that this will only occur in genetically predisposed individuals. However, people suffering from IBS who also have chronic stress are less likely to see their symptoms improve, which has led doctors to introduce stress management as a treatment for this syndrome. Meditation, yoga, and other relaxation exercises can decrease the frequency and severity of symptoms.

➤ Inflammatory Bowel Disease
Unlike those with IBS, people with inflammatory bowel disease (IBD) have chronic inflammation within their intestines that causes abdominal pain, diarrhea, rectal bleeding, and changes in appetite. Other organs such as the joints, skin, eyes, and bones can be damaged as well. Ulcerative colitis and Crohn's disease, both forms of IBD, are complex autoimmune conditions in which the immune system targets and attacks the tissues in its own body. Whereas ulcerative colitis involves mainly the large intestine, Crohn's disease can affect any part of the gut from the mouth to the anus. The cause of IBD is not well understood, and because it has phases of flare-ups and remission when the condition worsens and improves, patients are often under the continuing care of a gastroenterologist to manage their symptoms.

Studies have shown that stress, including chronic stress, adverse life events, and depression, increases the frequency of relapse in IBD. We know that stress hormones (cortisol and adrenaline) cause inflammation and that they create a vulnerable gut lining by decreasing blood supply, suppressing mucus production, and causing changes to the bacteria and acidity (pH) of the gut.[9] Often, harmful bacteria produce toxins that erode the lining. To defend itself from these attacks, the body sends in an army of immune cells to the lining. These cells burst, leaking histamine and other inflammatory chemicals into the gut. Eventually, this localized inflammation spreads throughout the body and becomes systemic.

We cannot say with certainty that negative mindsets cause IBD; however, we can link flare-ups of IBD to emotional stress. IBD currently has no known cure, so treatment addresses the inflammation and diarrhea and includes drugs such as steroids, anti-inflammatories, antispasmodics, and recently, prescribed biologics to reduce the symptoms. Stress management makes a significant difference when dealing with this condition.

Case Study: Joe

Joe was finishing his first year of university when he came to see me several years ago, complaining of severe diarrhea. We were both concerned that his situation, combined with weight loss and long-lasting and persistent colds and coughs, might indicate early inflammatory bowel disease. The local health clinic had offered drugs to stop the diarrhea and help with heartburn. However, no one had taken a full history or connected the dots to the root cause of the problem.

As we talked, it emerged that his mother was a cook in a local hospital and had made regular, healthy meals for Joe until he started university. The food in the residence cafeterias was not supplying the quality nutrients he needed nor was it very appetizing, so he often skipped meals and filled up with fast food instead. This change of diet, plus five to six cups of coffee during the day and a heavy increase of alcohol intake in the evenings, meant his gut lining was taking a beating. I conducted a few tests and found that he tested positive for harmful *H. pylori* bacteria, had white blood cells in his stool, and showed signs of dysbiosis.

While poor diet, too much alcohol, and irregular eating were big factors in why Joe developed diarrhea, the largest contributor was likely his emotional stress load. He was dealing with a recent relationship breakup and school assignments with tight deadlines. As expected, he was also having difficulty coping with painful and embarrassing bowel problems, which only added to his anxiety. There was a clear relationship between poor diet, high stress, and the onset of his symptoms. The first clue was the timing of his symptoms, which dated to the start of the academic year, his move away from home, and the subsequent breakup with his girlfriend.

Once the root cause became clear, so did the treatment. I started Joe on a complete 5R gut program (page 110), which removes abnormal gut flora and toxins, replaces them with healing foods and supplements, reinoculates the gut with healthy flora, regenerates the damaged villi and mucosal lining of the gut, and retains that healthy environment with a high-fiber diet. To address his immediate symptoms, such as diarrhea and pain, Joe received a prescription for antibiotics to treat *H. pylori*, the opportunistic bad bacteria in his gut. Next, he began to eat a largely plant-based diet with clean fats, small amounts of meat, and bone broth, and he eliminated alcohol and coffee to allow his gut lining to heal. Then he introduced probiotic foods like yogurt and other fermented foods (which contain gut-friendly bacteria such as lactobacillus and bifidobacterium) and supplements to heal the leaky junctions. He also began to practice stress management techniques. Within a few weeks of treatment, Joe was feeling better and his health continued to improve thereafter.

By the end of the summer, Joe was ready to go back to university. This time, he was armed with a thorough understanding of the mind-brain-body (gut) connection and tools to prevent his gut symptoms from recurring.

When the gut is compromised through inflammation, an overabundance of candida yeast,[10] and a shortage of good bacteria, it cannot produce serotonin (the "happy hormone"), which causes the body even more stress. And stressed people often consume more alcohol, coffee, sugary snacks, or takeout food to get a temporary "happiness high" to replace the lost serotonin. These choices cause more inflammation in the gut and the body.

➤ My Story

My gut was an intermittent source of medical issues even before my accident. When I was a first-year university student at age 17, I developed heartburn, which later turned into burning abdominal pain. After visiting the student health department many times and going through some tests, I was diagnosed with GERD and a possible peptic ulcer. Looking back, I realize that I put myself under extreme stress by taking three advanced science courses with labs, including chemistry.

I had never taken chemistry in high school and failed my first few exams in this course at university. This was a terrible blow to someone who had never failed a test! The harder I tried to learn the material, the more stressed I became. So overwhelming was the fear of failure that I drove myself to the brink of stress ulcers. A wise and caring professor took me aside and told me I wouldn't learn chemistry until I learned to relax and enjoy it. After a few sessions in his lab, witnessing some amazing chemical reactions and his pure passion for the science, I learned to relax and embrace the learning and not stress about getting an A on the exam. Miraculously, I passed his course with a solid B and not only that, I majored in pharmacy, which is largely chemistry based. I certainly wouldn't have predicted that outcome.

Following the accident, I took narcotic painkillers that caused severe constipation and forced me to use drugs to help promote bowel movements. These medications later wreaked havoc with my stomach lining, and my heartburn returned after years of being a non-issue. The stress and pain caused me anxiety and contributed to my gut dysfunction, as did the medications. After several years of dealing with gut issues, I became sensitive to certain foods, developed allergy symptoms, and had more colds and flus than I ever had before. But it wasn't until after my training in mind-body medicine that I made the profound association between poor gut health and a poor immune system.

I am much more aware of my gut health now and take good care of my gut lining by following the 5R gut program. I know how to regulate my stress hormones, avoid medications that disrupt the gut, and choose healthy foods that support my gut immune system. I know that my state of mind directly impacts my body and especially my gut.

HOW TO CULTIVATE A HEALTHY GUT MINDSET

Every aspect of our body function relies on our ability to digest properly. A relaxed gut absorbs nutrients and makes them widely available throughout the body. A well-functioning gut aids the immune system and does not initiate inflammation. A healthy gut manufactures serotonin, which calms us and can mean the difference between feeling lousy or well.

Learning to stimulate the vagus nerve is a crucial part of re-setting digestion. Communicating through the vagus nerve from the brain, the PNS applies the brakes to initiate our rest-and-digest response. When we feel safe, relaxed, and at rest, the PNS increases secretions and peristaltic movement within our gut and redirects blood flow there to allow more nutrients to be absorbed.

The gut and the brain work together to keep serotonin levels circulating and balanced in our blood. Neuroendocrine cells in the gut, called enterochromaffin cells, manufacture 80 to 85 percent of the serotonin in the body. Some immune cells and gut neurons manufacture it as well. In addition, some of our good gut bacteria stimulate the gut neurons to produce serotonin. In the brain, nerve cells called raphe neurons make serotonin. The chemical is molecularly identical whether the gut or the brain makes it, but the effect on each tissue is different. In the brain, serotonin or "the happy hormone" helps regulate appetite, cognition, mood, sexual behavior, and sleep. In the gut, serotonin helps contract our intestinal muscles and signals nausea or pain.

Eat a Healthy Diet

In the short term, eating a healthy diet is one of the most beneficial things you can do to combat stress and restore health. When we put nutritious food in our body, we are giving our cells the materials they need to grow, repair, and heal. We are putting fewer demands on our digestive system and our immune system to eliminate toxins and fight off disease. And as our gut has to work less hard, we begin to feel happier, lighter, and more energetic. What I like about the Institute for Functional Medicine's 5R gut program[11] is that it isn't just about removing foods from your diet. It's also about supporting your digestive system—your mind and body, in fact—with a healthy diet and a healthy attitude toward food and health. I use slightly different words with my patients, but the idea is the same.

➤ Heal and Repair with the 5R Gut Program

Doctors have long used the comprehensive 5R gut program to successfully reverse and heal a multitude of gut dysfunctions. I have followed it myself and recommended it to my patients, always with good results. Before you begin, do a gut health assessment (Appendix A) to see which areas of your gut (for example, upper gut, midgut, or lower bowels) are affected. If you have weight loss, diarrhea, blood or mucus in your stools, fever, chills, or muscle weakness, contact your health-care practitioner immediately. Whether you are experiencing these severe symptoms or not, discuss the 5R gut program with a medical professional to see if it can improve your overall health. You will be removing abnormal gut flora and toxins, replacing them with healing foods and supplements, repopulating the gut with healthy flora, regenerating the damaged villi and mucosal lining of the gut, and retaining that healthy environment with a high-fiber diet.

Remove. First, eliminate the things that irritate the gut. Clean up your diet by noticing symptoms shortly after you eat certain foods. In particular, pay attention to three categories of foods that can act as allergens and set off reactions in our gut without us being aware.

1. Irritants such as alcohol, caffeine, commercial dairy products, and refined carbs, such as high-fructose corn syrup, sugar, and wheat, all of which contribute to inflammation in the body.

2. Infectious agents such as giardia, yeast overgrowth, and parasites as well as *H. pylori*, all of which can grow out of control to cause acid reflux and heartburn. *H. pylori* infections can also cause chronic inflammation related to stomach cancer when untreated. It can be hard to tell if you've ingested one of these infectious agents, but diagnosis can be made with a breath test, blood test, or stool culture. If a test is positive, antibiotics are generally effective at getting rid of these agents but may also strip the gut of good bacteria.

3. Medications such as ibuprofen and aspirin, which are irritants to the gut. Avoid regular use of these drugs unless specified by a doctor.

Any or all of these foods, microorganisms, and medications can irritate the gut, but stressors, both physical and psychological, magnify the problem. They stimulate the fight-or-flight reaction, which impedes digestion.

Removing foods such as refined sugar, processed wheat, and commercial dairy from your diet and cutting out alcohol and caffeine for three to six weeks generally improves the gut health of most people. After that period, many people can reintroduce maple syrup, raw cane sugar, or dates; goat's milk or organic cow's milk; and whole grains or wheat alternatives to their diet. However, some people with high sensitivity to particular ingredients have to eliminate foods such as gluten, lectins, and beans from their diet in order to maintain a healthy gut.

If you continue to experience gut issues after cleaning up your diet, you may want to begin by keeping a food diary to see if you can note patterns between what you eat, when you eat it, and how you feel. Discuss your findings with your health-care practitioner. In certain cases, food allergy testing is warranted to confirm the specific foods that are causing gut distress.

Replace. When the gut is not working properly, secretions such as stomach acid, bile salts, and digestive enzymes diminish. As a result, we cannot properly digest food and use the micronutrients from the food we eat. The next step, therefore, is to recognize the symptoms of each deficiency so we can replace what is missing. Ask your health practitioner about completing a gut health assessment (Appendix A), so they can discuss and evaluate your symptoms and suggest some concrete solutions.

Repair. When ongoing irritation and inflammation break down the gut barrier, the junctions between them open, allowing toxins, bacteria, and undigested food to contact the sensitive membrane lining. The cells get shorter and they lose their protective armor of mucus. It is preferable that repair should occur with choosing the right foods, eliminating toxins, and reducing stress load. However, depending on the severity of symptoms, some people will require additional gut support to repair their gut. Most often, supplements (Appendix B) that heal the gut, such as glutamine or slippery elm, are used under the guidance of a health-care provider. Sometimes additional testing is required to rule out serious diseases. Use supplements under the guidance of a health-care practitioner.

Repopulate. The trillions of healthy bacteria in our microbiome detoxify our gut in addition to producing healthy mucus for our gut lining, essential vitamins for our body, and neurotransmitters such as serotonin for communication with the brain. When inflammation, poor diet, irritation, medication, or infection change the biochemistry of our gut, the healthy bacteria cannot survive and multiply; they become outnumbered by bad bacteria.

Eating fermented foods is a great way to repopulate the gut with good bacteria from natural probiotics such as bifidobacterium and lactobacillus. Fermentation occurs when foods containing sugar or starch are broken down by bacteria and yeast, and it's an ancient technique used to preserve food. Almost every culture contains some form of fermented food, whether it's pickles, yogurt, kimchi, or sauerkraut. Other examples include kombucha, kefir, and apple cider vinegar. As with any food, always read the label to check the serving size and sugar content.

Maintaining a diet rich in prebiotics (foods rich in fiber), such as artichokes, leeks, asparagus, garlic, and onions, is a good way to feed our healthy bacteria and promote their growth and activity in our gut. However, some health conditions, including IBS and IBD, may require commercial probiotics to help repopulate the gut with healthy bacteria. Look for human microflora multistrain bacteria that come as capsules or liquid cultures (Appendix B). Speak to your health-care practitioner, as high-potency probiotics may not be available off the shelf.

No matter how healthy your diet, some micronutrients are not in sufficient supply in food. In these cases, it can be helpful to take dietary supplements. For example, omega-3 fish oils (or flax) and vitamin D help support the immune system, and trace minerals such as magnesium support the gut and are often lacking in people with high stress. Some people require supplemental digestive enzymes as they age. Consult with your health-care practitioner before taking supplements or significantly changing your diet.

Relax/Rest. The most important R in the 5R program is relax, because digestion starts in the mind and optimum digestion happens when we are in a relaxed mental state. There is little point in spending hundreds of dollars on organic food and expensive gut supplements if we live in a constant state of anxiety. Only when we are at rest and in a relaxed state is the blood flow directed back to the miles of gut tissue and do the muscles for contractions and secretions for digestion work more effectively. Thus, we must be mindful when we eat and employ all our stress-reduction techniques to remain calm and relaxed (see the Breath, Mind, Word Method, page 82).

←——→

TRY THESE ADDITIONAL STEPS to feed your gut for optimum health.

➤ Break the Cycle of Emotional Eating

To create a healthy gut mindset, we need to understand the connection between our mind, our brain, and our gut. *The mind forms a belief; the brain embeds it; the body executes it.* At the root of our emotions and habits are events we have internalized. We associate these subconscious memories with deeper emotions and together they form beliefs about food and create our mindset.

We learned from Russian physiologist Ivan Pavlov's conditioning experiment with dogs[12] that when he rang a bell every time he fed the dog some meat, the dog learned to associate the bell ringing with food. It wasn't the meat itself that caused the dog to salivate; it was the *thought* of meat that caused the salivation response. In the same way, our emotions condition our response to food at a very early age. The mere sight, sound, smell, or touch of food triggers a response in the mind, meaning that digestion begins in the mind and not in the mouth.

Do you have fond memories of baking bread with your grandmother on a rainy day? Or gathering around the table with friends and family for turkey or matzo or dim sum or samosas on festive occasions? Or do you have bad memories of being forced to eat brussels sprouts or natto or some other food you didn't like? Our brain forms pathways of conditioning and patterns of associations with food. Thanks to our limbic system, thinking about a food we associate with an emotion elicits the same digestive juices as eating that food.

Part of cultivating a healthy gut mindset is being aware of emotional eating. Remember, upgrade your inner dialogue (page 28). We eat more when we are bored, anxious, or upset. For example, exam stress, poor diet, and binge drinking after exams create a perfect storm for gut problems. It isn't uncommon for university students to be treated for ulcers or GERD, especially during or after exams. To turn these impacts around, the first thing to do is note our automatic eating habits and food choices. Remember, our brain prioritizes survival, not happiness. To fend off a predator or escape danger, we need quick energy, which is why the brain is hardwired to locate and home in on sugar snacks. Simple sugars—like chocolate, candy, and pastries—are an instant source of energy. The key to cultivating a healthy relationship with food, and by extension our gut, is to consciously write the program. (See Tap into Your Conscious Brain, page 55.) Instead of living to eat (subconscious), we need to focus on eating to live (conscious). Changing our beliefs changes our actions. Instead of automatically reaching for the chocolate cake, we might consciously choose fresh fruit instead.

When we make up our mind, we are more able to stay on course and get the results we signed up for. When we create a conscious mindset for a healthy lifestyle, we are able to override the automatic habits that lead us to the cupboard or the fridge and the negative internal dialogue (often, "I am not _____ enough," or "If only I were _____ ") that keeps us on the same fight-or-flight pathway as if there were a tiger on our tail. This is the connection between emotional eating and food. Not only do we short-circuit the impulse to eat the chocolate cake (because our cortisol made us do it), we prevent the resulting emotional trigger—the guilt—that releases more cortisol into the body and perpetuates the cycle.

➤ Choose and Eat Your Food Mindfully
Every food you select is a decision, conscious or subconscious. Most often we choose foods mindlessly, giving in to our senses,

mental associations, and automatic habits. To make healthy choices an automatic habit, stay aware of what you eat and be fully present while eating. For example, if you find yourself eating a bag of chips, ask yourself whether you consciously chose it to feed your hunger or whether you are mindlessly emptying the bag because you're anxious or bored. After you have mindfully chosen the food (hopefully not chips), use all of your senses to experience it.

Follow these four steps:

1. *Observe the state of your body.* Is your stomach rumbling? Is your energy low? Consider whether you are hungry or whether something else is causing these sensations.

2. *Be fully present.* Turn off the TV, unplug your phone, sit down, and focus on who you are with and what you are doing.

3. *Take note of the food.* Breathe in its aroma, savor its flavor, and feel its texture in your mouth.

4. *Eat without judgment.* Observe the inner dialogue that runs as you savor your food. Are you feeling guilt? Are rigid rules popping into your head? If so, be self-compassionate.

Chew slowly and purposefully (Practice Mindfulness, page 31). Stay calm and relaxed to stimulate the vagus nerve and engage the brakes in your digestive system. Remember that to digest you must be at rest! Use the BMW meditation to re-set your ANS through deep, controlled breath (page 82). Eating mindfully has proven benefits such as weight loss and an improved psychological relationship with food, and the food actually tastes better too.

Some people find apps useful for mindful eating. For example, Am I Hungry? and Mindful Eating Tracker can help guide your decision-making process around eating, track your hunger and thirst, and help you to eat mindfully.

➤ Increase the Frequency and Intensity of Your Exercise

We know a good cardio workout makes you hungry. More than that, exercise has two main benefits. First, it sends oxygen-rich blood to the vessels that nourish the vital supporting organs of digestion such as the liver, pancreas, and kidneys. Once you return to a normal resting heart rate, the blood flow to your digestive system is redirected to the miles and miles of blood vessels in the gut lining. People often find that exercise also helps them have regular bowel movements and expel gas. Second, exercise reduces the stress hormones circulating in the blood. With less cortisol coursing through the body, homeostasis returns. The PNS prompts the digestive system, and the body grows, repairs, heals, and eliminates waste. For more on this subject, see Exercise Your Muscles (page 143).

The Benefits of a Healthy Gut

In the United States alone, more than 70 million people suffer with some form of gastrointestinal disorder and many more experience chronic disease that is associated with gut dysfunction. Research suggests that some of these people perceive pain more acutely than other people do because their brains are more responsive to pain signals from the GI tract. Stress can make the existing pain seem even worse. And stress and pain in the gut can be carried through the enteric nervous system to the brain, where it contributes to anxiety and depression.[13]

Therefore, a healthy gut contributes to overall physical, emotional, and mental health more than just about any other system in the body.

We know that information travels from the gut to the brain along nerve pathways in the blink of an eye, much quicker than information relayed via more traditional hormonal networks.[14] While this signaling system may have developed to detect toxins in the gut and relay that information immediately to the brain so the body can activate its defense units, this system also seems to affect mood. At a basic level, this pathway may be the reason that eating makes us feel good. We also know that particular bacteria from the gut microbiome stimulate gut endocrine cells to produce serotonin. This serotonin produced in the gut shows up in the colon—where it helps control peristalsis and digestion—and it is also picked up by blood platelets and circulated to all parts of the body except the brain. Serotonin is linked to positive mood, lower levels of anxiety and depression, better sleep, and improved brain function.

CONCLUSION

"Let food be thy medicine," said Hippocrates, the father of medicine, many years ago. While nutrition is essential, we cannot have a healthy gut unless we have a healthy mind. Our brain is sending signals to the gut 24/7 from the moment we are born until the moment we die. Regardless of whether we are awake, asleep, or even unconscious, messages are being sent and received. This crosstalk has an impact on our mood, how we make decisions, and even how much we eat. The key is to understand that our mind can help regulate our gut function to achieve optimal health. When we live in perpetual fear or with chronic negativity, stress hormones impair the blood flow to the gut, shut down secretions from the gut to conserve energy, and put digestion on hold until we perceive safety. Therefore, to have proper digestion, we must be in a relaxed state. Remember, rest and digest!

Healthy digestion starts in the mind. Organic groceries, good-quality vitamins, and probiotics help keep our gut healthy—but only when we consume these in a positive state of mind. Keep both your mind and your gut healthy and it will pay enormous dividends to your overall physical, emotional, and mental well-being.

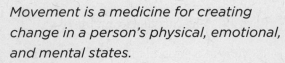

5.

Mind Your Movement

Movement is a medicine for creating change in a person's physical, emotional, and mental states.
Carol Welch

SELF-ASSESSMENT

How well do you use movement to cope with stress? Exercise relieves stress by boosting chemicals that relax and nourish the brain. Physical activity improves blood flow to all our organs and tissues, making them resilient to stress. Most people know that exercise is good for the body but they are too stressed, distracted, or busy to fit it into their routine. Chronic stress is associated with diminished activity level, weight gain, and a long list of medical problems that go along with being sedentary.

Do you:

· avoid activity?

· park close to the store to avoid walking as far?

· get short of breath easily?

- complain of fatigue and low mood?

- have poor sleep habits?

- have a high resting heart rate (over 100 beats per minute)?

- get injured easily while participating in physical activity?

- get achy muscles even after a small amount of physical activity?

- experience stiff joints?

- have difficulty carrying heavy objects?

Movement is integral to being alive, and as humans we have evolved and adapted to our environment because we move effectively. At the most basic level, we have survived as a species because our mobility system has allowed us to access food rather than become food. A pregnant woman cannot contain her excitement when she feels her baby's first movement. That distinctive flutter from her uterus signals life and well-being for her unborn child. If movement stops, she knows something is wrong. As our organs develop, all our body systems become sensitive to movement and learn to integrate, allowing our body to function as one unit.

In past generations, people moved from sunup to sundown. They hunted and gathered, felled trees for shelter, mined metals for trade and tools, worked the land for food. Industrialization brought automation and technology, and now many of us schedule special exercise time at the gym because we spend our days sitting at desks staring into computer screens. "Sitting is the new smoking," read headlines, and the fine print adds that we stew and stress while we sit. It's a double whammy. Prolonged sitting is not good for our body, but stressing while sitting is even worse. Stress hormones were designed to make us move, just as they cause animals to fight or flee in threatening situations. Yet when we are sedentary, these same hormones cause inflammation instead. One of the common risk factors for heart disease, breast cancer, and even Alzheimer's disease is inactivity. In contrast, people who incorporate physical activity into their daily life are more adaptable and resilient to physical and emotional stress.

Why are some people motivated to exercise while others, despite knowing about the benefits of movement, are not? The answer is mindset. To hardwire healthy habits of movement so they become second nature, we need to harness the power of the subconscious mind. Exercise is a major tool for fighting stress and creating resilience, and the quicker we learn to program our mind to embrace this idea, the better off we will be.

EXERCISE 101

Kinesiology—or exercise science—is the study of movement, and it draws on research in biomechanics, anatomy, physiology, psychology, and neuroscience. By understanding how and why the body moves, we can optimize its ability to carry out these functions. For elite athletes, more efficient movement can mean the difference between a winning performance and chronic injury. For most of us, regular movement helps our body become strong and resilient, so we can easily adapt to different conditions to prevent injury and disease. Our musculoskeletal system comprises muscles, bones, tendons, and ligaments as well as all the other connective tissues and joints that hold it together (Figure 5.1). Its main function is to support the body, protect vital organs, and allow activity and movement.

Movement seems to be very simple and mechanistic, yet it requires the coordination of many different systems in the body. The three main systems that exert their control over the musculoskeletal system are the nervous, circulatory, and respiratory systems. Together they allow the brain and nerves to carefully coordinate and orchestrate communication for purposeful movement while ensuring adequate blood supply and oxygen, especially during exercise.

Exercise is the regular, repeated, and targeted movement of different muscles in the body. Exercise prepares our heart to adapt when stress causes it to beat fast and fear urges us to run away. Exercise prepares our arms and legs to adapt when stress causes us to push away heavy objects to get out of harm's way. Exercise prepares our tendons and ligaments to adapt when we encounter uneven ground and rebalance to prevent a fall. So when we talk about exercise, we're talking about aerobic (cardio), anaerobic (strength building), and flexibility (stretching) activities.

Aerobic exercise trains our cardiac muscle (heart) and the smooth muscles in our respiratory passages and blood vessels. Intense workouts such as running and interval training push oxygen to the brain and to all the small blood vessels in the body.

Anaerobic exercise trains the skeletal muscles and the tendons and ligaments. More than 600 of these muscles create movement in the body, yet this lean muscle mass naturally decreases with age and is replaced by fat. So anaerobic exercise—also known as muscle strengthening, progressive muscle resistance, or weight training—pushes blood to these muscles, which helps to maintain and even increase their mass. Increased muscle mass translates to increased bone mass.

Flexibility exercises train our skeletal muscles, tendons, ligaments, and bones. Stretching, such as yoga, tai chi, and qigong, works the muscles and the fascia and ligaments that hold everything together, pushing blood to all these parts to improve balance, strength, and flexibility.

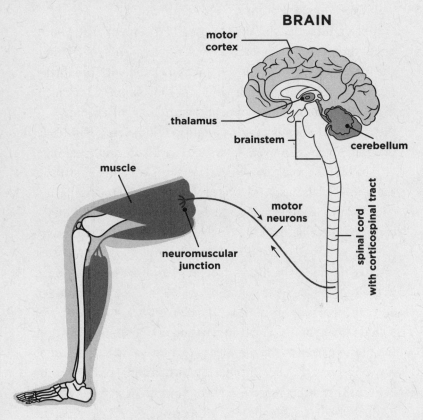

Figure 5.1. The musculoskeletal system

Many research studies have also established that aerobic exercise improves the flow of blood in the brain and enhances the function of many neurotransmitters involved in cognitive functioning. So movement is not just good for our body, it is also crucial in maintaining our brain function, especially as we age. To understand why, it helps to understand how muscle movement works.

Voluntary and Involuntary Movement

Our brain directly controls almost all movement in the body, either through the autonomic nervous system (ANS) or through the motor system. The movement associated with breathing, heart function, circulation, and other *involuntary* actions is directed by the ANS. A region of the cerebral cortex known as the motor area sends motor signals to the skeletal muscles to produce *voluntary* movements, such as walking and speaking.

The brain's motor (movement) system is contained mostly in the frontal lobes. It starts with premotor areas, for planning and coordinating complex movements, and ends with the primary motor cortex, where the final instructions are sent down the spinal cord to cause contraction and movement of specific muscles. Just like the neural pathways in other parts of the body, the ones in the motor system are bidirectional. Sensors in the muscles and other parts of the peripheral nervous system send sensory signals to the brain. The transmission of a motor signal from the motor cortex to the muscles is carried out in two different ways: by direct transfer through the corticospinal tract to motor neurons that direct muscle fibers or by indirect transfer via the cerebellum, basal ganglia, and various nuclei of the brainstem to the motor neurons (Figure 5.1).

In this indirect system, the message relay station is the thalamus. This mass of gray matter at the base of the brainstem receives both sensory and motor signals and sends them to the cerebral cortex, which delegates them to the appropriate area of the brain for processing. For example, the cerebellum helps coordinate movement by comparing the action you wanted with the action you're doing, and it corrects the movement if there is a problem. It is also involved in acquiring motor skills such as learning to ride a bike. The basal ganglia are involved in controlling complex patterns of movements, including balance.

Muscles move on commands from the brain. The only way the brain connects to muscles is through nerve cells called motor neurons in the spinal cord. Each motor neuron connects to just one muscle, say the quadriceps at the front of your upper thigh that extends your leg. When a motor neuron fires, it sends a chemical impulse along its long, thin axon to the muscle. At the neuromuscular junction—the site where motor neurons and muscle cells communicate—the impulse causes the release of a neurotransmitter that bridges the space between the two cells and sends forward the message. Receptors on the muscle cell then cause the muscle fibers to ratchet past each other, overlapping each other more, so that the muscle gets shorter and fatter. Simply stated, the muscle contracts. When the impulse from the nerve stops, the muscle fibers slide back to their original position and the contraction ends.

A muscle cell is unique among cells in our body because it contains many nuclei. As we exercise, the muscle fibers grow and nuclei can multiply, and these nuclei remain throughout our lives whether the cell is in active use or not. In fact, our muscle cells have extraordinary memory capabilities: they will remember the size and shape of an exercised muscle even if we stop exercising. This is why kids who grow up playing sports and then stop have an easier time getting fit later in life—their muscle cells recall the previous conditioning and quickly organize themselves to return to their earlier fitness. Our muscle cells can also memorize complex tasks requiring extensive muscle coordination. They will remember the movements needed to ride a bike or play a musical instrument even if we go many years without doing them.

Our muscles also communicate with the brain. In fact, our brain health is dependent on signals sent by large muscles to the brain, which is why people with muscle atrophy, such as in multiple sclerosis and motor neuron disease, see rapid overall health declines.[1] The same is true of patients confined to bed or astronauts in space whose large muscles bear no weight. Not only do they experience muscle loss, their body chemistry changes at a cellular level and may impair their balance. Weight-bearing exercises, in particular, send signals to the neural cells in the brain to promote new growth and repair. It is theorized that a lack of movement (especially aerobic exercise) reduces the amount of oxygen to the brain's mitochondria, which are vital for energy and metabolism.

This bidirectional flow of information between the brain and the musculoskeletal system highlights the brain's ability to respond to different conditions. It is helpful to recognize the brain as both "plastic and dynamic," in a constant state of flux and kinetic growth. That growth can come from physical stimulus such as exercise, but it can also be affected by mental or emotional activity. For example, when we are sad, depressed, or unhappy, these emotions impact how much we move and how we hold our body. Movement is biologically hardwired into our system as a cue to wake up and pay attention. It sends signals to our brain to become aware of what is surrounding us, calls us to action, makes us more alert to decisions that have to be made, opportunities that are available, and threats that need to be avoided. We see how the mind (thoughts) impact our brain

(ANS, motor systems, limbic system) and how it causes lack of movement. By the same token, we see how our body also sends signals to our brain to keep it functioning at its optimal capacity.

In his book *Spark*, John Ratey summarized the connection between exercise and the brain: "The more complex the movements, the more complex the synaptic connections. And even though these circuits are created through movement, they can be recruited by other areas and used for thinking... The prefrontal cortex will co-opt the mental power of the physical skills and apply it to other situations."[2] In other words, exercise doesn't just send oxygen to the brain so it can create new neurons, it challenges those neurons to make new connections. By putting those new brain cells to use, it creates patterns of sensation and response that can be used throughout the body.

Movement as a Stimulus for Body Integration and Resilience

We know that muscles move when signals from the brain produce electrical changes in muscle cells. When the nervous system signals skeletal muscle to contract, groups of these muscles work together to move our body. These signals and movements are nearly involuntary, but not quite. That is, we need to consciously decide to move our arms and legs, for example, but we don't need to concentrate on each individual muscle when moving them. Our cardiac muscle and the smooth muscles in our respiratory system and blood vessels are completely involuntary, though hormones and stimuli from the nervous system can affect their rhythm, such as increasing heart rate when we're scared.

Stress revs up the gas, forcing all the systems in the body to communicate closely and organize more efficiently for survival.

Similarly, exercise is an excellent way to increase endurance, stamina, and strength because it forces the body's physiological systems to communicate better, and this body integration makes us stronger both mentally and physically. We rarely talk about this benefit of body integration as an advantage for survival for those who exercise compared with those who remain sedentary.

Our external environment is constantly changing, and being physically adaptable is a key trait to withstand stress. Integrating the body's communication systems gives us an edge because it allows us to respond faster and more efficiently to stress, which gives us greater resilience and is invaluable for increasing our longevity. Resilience means having the capacity to withstand pressure or recover quickly from difficult circumstances without breaking. Exercise makes us resilient!

Movement as the Impetus for Muscle Cell Growth

Skeletal muscle makes up about 40 percent of the body (smooth and cardiac muscle make up another 5 to 10 percent). While the brain communicates with our muscle cells, we also know these cells—in fact, all cells in the body—can communicate internally or with other cells. Cell-signaling theory describes the complex network needed to send and receive these messages. In essence, an army of signaling molecules (chemical compounds, electrical impulses, or mechanical stimuli) spreads the message across and between cells by seeking targets (receptors) that receive the initial signal. With the message received, the cell then responds by carrying out the instruction or by initiating a message of its own.

Movement from the body initiates just this kind of cell signaling. For example, when skeletal muscle cells are stretched—deformed or damaged by exercise—calcium ions flood into the muscle cell. This mechanical signal, the flux of calcium ions, triggers a number of cell-signaling pathways inside the muscle, including hormones responsible for muscle growth. Hormones are a chemical signal; they travel through the bloodstream to the brain and other tissues with a message that the skeletal muscle cells need to grow, multiply, and be renewed.

As sophisticated and complex as this two-way information highway is, the brain sends only two messages through our nervous system: grow or decay. In a muscle that moves regularly, communication proteins signal the brain and other tissues in the body that it needs nutrients to repair minor tears and grow stronger. If there is no movement in a muscle—say, if you hurt your calf muscle and cannot use it—it does not produce communication proteins, and the brain reads the lack of signals as a sign of "decay" or deconditioning. The efficient brain sees no point in sending blood supply and nutrients to an area that is not being used, and the muscle begins to atrophy. This is cell-signaling theory in action.

We've all heard the expression "use it or lose it," and this principle exactly describes how the brain allocates nutrients and blood supply. The brain requires a signal from the muscles that they are indeed alive and well and being used. So, common medical practice now has athletes moving as soon as possible after an injury, even if it is only passive movement, when someone else—such as a physiotherapist—is moving the limb for you. Even surgeons who replace knee joints get their patients moving a day after the surgery. Similarly, when we are sedentary, we are telling our brain that our muscles are not being used, to preserve the nutrients and energy for something else or store them for future use. The more sedentary we are, the higher the risk of sarcopenia, or muscle loss. Sarcopenia occurs with aging or lack of use and puts us at a higher risk for falling and fractures, especially if our bones are soft. It is also a big predictor of poor aging and bone health.

With aging, we often measure a decrease in the rate of muscle fiber contractions, letting the brain know the muscles are not being used. The brain, in its efficient manner of delegating energy resources, sends signals communicating "decay." This is very common in the elderly who do not remain active. If we want to age well, we need to keep moving as much as we can for as long as we can so our muscles continue to get a "grow" signal from the brain, thereby ensuring a good supply of nerves and blood vessels to maintain muscle mass. Remember, there are two basic signals from the brain to muscles: "grow" or "decay." It's up to you to remain active so you continue to receive grow signals . . . Who wants to decay?

STRESS HORMONES AND RESTRICTED MOVEMENT

Muscle memory helps our cells remember proper conditioning and complex movements, but if we injure ourselves, the muscles also remember the pain associated with that injury so we don't reinjure ourselves in the same way. Physically injured muscles are often inflamed and in pain, thus they become more constricted and tense. Constant tension in the muscles, even if they are not inflamed, leads to a reduced range of motion or lack of mobility. Muscles memorize the reduced range of motion, which results in body stiffness and deconditioning. So sitting for long periods of time—whether working on a computer or playing games on your phone or another device—can cause muscle tension. But so too can an emotional memory.

Our bodies have a threshold for handling stress, and trauma results when an experience exceeds our ability to cope with its consequences. For example, a sudden car accident overloads the nervous system as the body goes into instinctive fight-or-flight mode. As it revs up the gas, it stores the traumatic energy in the muscles, organs, and fibrous connective tissues around them (fascia). If the body experiences whiplash, for example, this energy might be stored in the muscles and fascia of the neck, spine, and back. If the impact causes an injury to the arm, this energy might be stored in the muscles and fascia of the neck, shoulder, and bicep. This is a protective mechanism, and until we release this energy, it can lead to muscle pain and fatigue.

Pain that lasts longer than normal for natural healing becomes chronic. The pain signals are being sent to the brain repeatedly and along the same pathway that signals danger. The ANS therefore interprets pain as danger and sends out cortisol and adrenaline to initiate the fight-or-flight reaction. Sometimes, these pathways become so rehearsed that they respond automatically even after the physical wounds have healed.

While stress can lead to illness, illness can also lead to stress. Physical pain, missed activities, feelings of isolation, and other costs that come with a chronic illness result in stress.

How Stress Affects Our Movement

Ample data exists on the benefits of activity to relieve stress, anxiety, and depression. Fewer studies look at the restrictions that stress places on movement. However, just as chronic stress is associated with higher rates of smoking, alcohol and drug use, and overeating, it also appears to impede our ability to make healthy choices about physical activity in general.[3] Researchers conclude that in some cases, people with chronic stress choose to be less active or inactive because they have little time or do not prioritize exercise. In other cases, the brain seems to feel it is a "waste of time" to pursue a physical activity when the body is in crisis. However, how active a person is when stressed seems to be more related to their level of activity before the stress load. If they were regular exercisers before stress, they seem to increase activity at times of increased stress. If they were not regular exercisers, they tend to use stress as an excuse to avoid physical activity.

Chronically elevated cortisol levels impair protein synthesis, which is the cornerstone of developing muscle mass. We know that lack of physical activity leads to muscle loss by itself, but when combined with elevated cortisol, that effect seems to be greater. Cortisol has a catabolic effect on muscle tissue, meaning that the tissue breaks down. A study showed that prolonged exposure to cortisol negatively impacts the recovery of muscle function. Higher levels of cortisol also have a strong correlation to central fat obesity (also called visceral fat), which is fat accumulation around the belly. Not only do I see in practice that more stress hormones lead to more body fat, but research shows that visceral body fat is associated with a whole host of chronic diseases such as type 2 diabetes and heart disease. Building muscle and losing fat is more difficult while under stress, and unchecked cortisol lowers our level of activity, reduces our muscle recovery, and changes our body composition. Several conditions are associated with limited movement.

➤ Muscle Tension and Joint Stiffness

When we sit in one position for too long, it affects the range of motion of certain joints, which were designed to move. Our joints are hinges designed to improve agility and weight bearing.

Exercise helps the joints that connect bones to stay lubricated, whereas sitting still causes the joints to stiffen and increases inflammation. Our muscles need us to use them to remain conditioned. We need to stretch and stimulate our fascia, ligaments, and tendons. More importantly, these tissues need to work together to create smooth musculoskeletal integration. Sitting still causes all of these mechanical working parts to stiffen up and become inflamed.

Many people report neck, shoulder, and back pain after working at their desk every day. We weren't meant to sit at a desk or punch keys for hours at a time. To avoid stiffness and injury—including repetitive strain injuries—our spine should be mobile and flexible and needs to change positions, as do all of our body parts. Muscle tension is also commonly associated with anxiety and stress, which causes the muscles to remain clenched (contracted) for long periods of time. Be sure to build breaks into your workday so you can get up, move around, and de-stress. Try to vary your working position by introducing a standing or running desk or doing tasks away from a desk.

➤ Psychomotor Retardation

Chronic stress is often associated with low mood. Prolonged and pervasive sadness, grief, and depression send signals to our motor cortex to slow down body movements and reflexes, including speech, facial expressions, and agility.[4] In extreme cases of depression, this psychomotor retardation can cause people to go into a catatonic state in which they just curl up and are unable to will themselves to move. Cortisol may be interfering with dopamine transmission in the brain so the command center has "checked out" or gone offline. Using movement and exercise to trigger the brain to normal activity is key to re-establishing regular function. With movement, we begin to stimulate electrical circuits that involve the limbic and motor pathway systems. Movement helps circulate oxygenated blood in these highly connected systems, which can reactivate networks that were temporarily shut down.

➤ Strains, Sprains, and Other Injuries

Many people become overzealous and ambitious with exercise and end up with injuries that cause more stress. The key to avoiding injury is to build up slowly. If you have an injury or setback, think of it as an obstacle to overcome. For example, one of my patients wanted to lose weight for her upcoming reunion, and I wanted her to reduce her risk for disease, for better health. I outlined the benefits of exercise, and she decided to start a Zumba dance class. However, after only the second class, she injured her ankle and required a walking cast. She returned to my office quite deflated. She had convinced herself that the ankle injury meant she couldn't walk or do any other exercise in case she caused further injury. When I suggested swimming, she was surprised. She hadn't thought of it, because in her mind, the ankle injury and cast meant "rest" the whole body.

Injuries and setbacks can cause a lot of muscle deconditioning, so check with your physiotherapist or health-care provider to see what activities will not further damage the injured area. Chair yoga, stretching, and swimming are often good alternatives when you hit a roadblock with activities that involve weight bearing. Be creative and find a way around the obstacle rather than finding ways to stay sedentary.

➤ Insulin Resistance and Weight Gain

When the body does not or cannot move naturally and regularly, a whole constellation of ill health and disease follows, including insulin resistance, weight gain, and obesity. As a physician, I recognize that diet and exercise are extremely important tools for weight loss; however, it is also vital to address the role of stress hormones. When stress (both overt and covert) is constant, prolonged, and excessive, our cortisol levels go up. Cortisol induces insulin resistance, which is a primary cause of abdominal fat and weight gain. When insulin does not work properly, it creates an imbalance in blood sugars that translates to fat deposits. More recently we have also discovered that other hormones involved with hunger and satiety—such as leptin, ghrelin, and adiponectin—play a part in the obesity cycle. Cortisol also influences how they work: we know that stressed individuals crave more sugar and stimulants.

Those who are sedentary also tend to consume high-sugar drinks and alcoholic beverages (beer, pop, juices), higher-carbohydrate foods, and sweets, all of which pave the way for obesity. Inactivity adds to the risk of higher blood sugars, and even for those at a healthy weight, being parked in a chair for too long increases the risk of diabetes and higher cholesterol. In Germany, people who logged the most sitting time also had higher rates of colon, endometrial, and lung cancer.[5] "Skinny-fat" people, who are not overweight but have a higher proportion of fat than muscle, still need to exercise!

The visceral fat that develops around the middle works against the body by producing more chemicals of inflammation. Tissues that are chronically inflamed create chemicals that attack cells, causing DNA damage.[6] Worst of all, excess fat tissue can produce toxic hormones that lead to more inflammation and cell proliferation. It is a vicious cycle.

➤ Muscle Wasting (Sarcopenia)

Skeletal muscle mass declines naturally with age, but inactivity expedites the process. We usually begin to lose mass as early as age 40 and may lose as much as half of our muscle mass by age 70—by which time the fat and fibrous tissue that replace our original fibers make our muscles look like a well-marbled steak! This muscle wasting, or sarcopenia, can lead to poor balance and falls, and it often precedes osteopenia (bone thinning), which later progresses to osteoporosis (softening of the bones). Sarcopenia is associated with insulin resistance and fatigue and can limit our independence. However, by watching how we exercise and what we eat, we can slow down muscle loss and even reverse it!

➤ Chronic Muscle Pain

We know physical trauma resulting from a motor vehicle accident or a physical assault engages the fight-or-flight system into a full-alarm state, and that the brain gets busy consolidating all the cues around the trauma so we never forget it. The amygdala and the associated limbic system create neural pathways that turn on "hypervigilance," with the result that we become extremely sensitized to anything that resembles the trauma. The actual event is long over, but the hypervigilance—and sometimes the memory of the traumatic pain—lasts well beyond the original incident.

The short-term memory of the trauma gets transported to the hippocampus, where we store it and assign emotions to it for the long term. For example, we store the smell, sound, taste, texture, and visual records remotely associated with the event in that consolidated memory. If we don't address and properly process the physical or emotional trauma early on, we may develop post-traumatic stress disorder (PTSD) and chronic pain. Hypersensitivity may lead us to notice nearly every physical sensation in our body. And any of those subconscious sensory memories associated with the trauma may trigger a visceral response, re-creating and amplifying in our body the pain associated with the original trauma. When that response is triggered repeatedly and persistently, the pain becomes chronic. A similar effect is at work among patients who have lost a limb and experience "phantom pain," a feeling of pain in the absent limb. Neuroscience explains that the brain generates the pain as if the limb exists, likely drawing on its muscle memory and disregulating the ANS.

➤ My Story

After my car accident, I underwent several surgeries and began physical therapy to treat bone, muscle, and nerve injuries. Despite these interventions, I experienced uncontrollable neck and shoulder pain, which became constant and debilitating. I couldn't sleep properly, and a simple, repetitive activity such as drying my hair or emptying the dishwasher would cause flare-ups of pain. I experienced pain both from nerves compressed by scar tissue (neurological) and from muscle tissue damaged in the accident (muscular), and I often required medications to control it so I could function. On X-rays there were no findings, which is not unusual since soft tissue injury and nerve impingement are difficult to visualize on X-ray, but the pain continued.

Only a few months had passed since the accident, but I became anxious because it was sometimes hard to control the pain and I worried about whether this was my new reality. The side effects of the prescriptions were gradual at first—some constipation and heartburn—but they later progressed to nausea and abdominal pain. My gut was not happy, and neither was I. After months of the same, I became depressed, not realizing how much impact pain and anxiety were having on my emotional state. Some days, nothing I tried gave me lasting relief. My right arm felt heavy, full of pins and needles, and often turned color due to compressed blood vessels.

Several years later, I was diagnosed with thoracic outlet syndrome and had surgery to free up the blood vessels and nerves caught in the scar tissue from the injury. With little sleep, constant pain, and no energy to exercise, my muscles became quite deconditioned, especially in my right hand and arm. My capacity to exercise was limited by pain, stiffness, and the resulting deconditioned muscles I was not using. On my "good" days, I was motivated to do some minimal stretching or walking, which left me out of breath and often in more pain. It was a vicious cycle that I knew I had to break.

Not being able to play ball with my children or engage with them physically was a terrible loss. I made up my mind to gradually increase exercise every day: I began to swim, stretch, and do yoga. It took years of physiotherapy, massage, and other treatments to improve my range of motion and slowly build up muscle again. The most profound change came when I began to use mindfulness-based breathing techniques to address pain. Fast-forward to my current state. It's as if I have a new body. I exercise daily, have much better range of motion, and feel so much stronger. Our body takes direction from our mind, and if we can tap into that program we can often heal and repair our muscle, bone, and fascia trauma. The mind has to collaborate with the brain and the body.

Lack of movement—whether from stress or inactivity—profoundly affects our mood. Feeling sad? Blame your chair! An Australian study showed that men who sat at their desks for over six hours a day had more psychological distress (nervousness, restlessness, fatigue, and feelings of hopelessness) than men who sat for only three hours a day.[7] Video games and TV, considered by many as favorite pastimes, may be detrimental to our mood and ability to connect with others. Heavy doses of technology are associated with higher rates of depression and suicide in teens.[8]

Being sedentary also destroys our sex drive. Many people complain they are simply too tired to have sex. If they have to choose between sleep or sex, sleep usually wins. Fit people feel better about their body image and want to engage in intimate activity, and they typically have better hormone function that supports it. A Harvard study found that men who had larger bellies had more erectile dysfunction and a lower sperm count.[9] Who would have thought exercise level affected the little swimmers?

Ironically, inactivity also greatly affects our ability to achieve deep, restorative sleep. People who exercise regularly report less insomnia, and we all know how beneficial a good night's sleep can be for our overall health.

HOW TO CULTIVATE A HEALTHY MOVEMENT MINDSET

Why do some people embrace exercise as second nature and others loathe it and treat it as punishment? This question comes up often in my practice, and I find it rather interesting. Our current "automatic, push-button" lifestyle plays a huge role, but the real answer is multifactorial. It may have something to do with having a mindset of movement. Childhood experiences such as outdoor play, parental role models, physical abilities, habit, and motivation help shape an individual's mindset about exercise that lasts a lifetime. Caregivers influence what a child perceives, believes, and achieves, along with the activity-related experiences the child has with those caregivers.

In my experience, one of the most important determinants of a person's activity level has more to do with deeply embedded beliefs and expectations about the potential benefits for their health. A core belief that exercise is good, combined with the confidence of knowing that exercise can make a positive difference to health, is vital for habitual movement. This belief helps form a person's overall attitude and behavior related to exercise, and it subconsciously differentiates those with a healthy movement mindset—the "active avocados"—from the "couch potatoes."

If you can move but think exercise is too difficult, embarrassing, painful, time consuming, or exhausting, perhaps you have locked into a fixed negative mindset about exercise. Your subconscious beliefs may be consistent with your lack of activity. Alternatively, you may exercise because you believe it helps to keep you fit and healthy (and you value that) and it makes you feel good. You have a pro-activity, positive mindset and consider exercise fun and a source of stress relief.

An interesting study done in 2010 at Penn State University used pedometers to measure the activity level of students.[10] Students with a positive attitude about exercise tended to move more frequently. They were the kids who took the stairs, didn't hesitate to walk to classes that were far away, and even parked their cars farther from campus so they could increase their step counts. Those with a negative attitude about exercise had substantially lower counts on their pedometers. Their subconscious program didn't motivate them to move as much or to take part in active behaviors. A profound relationship exists between mindset, exercise, and other health-related habits.[11]

Other factors may undermine an exercise mindset. Often, being overweight creates a mindset of being trapped and lacking control. Imagine trying numerous diets and exercise gizmos from infomercials and joining gyms only to lose weight initially and then gain it back (the yo-yo effect). Psychologically, these experiences of repeated failure lead to feelings of being stuck fat forever, reinforcing negative attitudes about exercise.

An honest self-appraisal of your mindset is a great place to start if you are less active. You can change negative beliefs and habits around exercise, and the first step is creating an awareness. We need to remind ourselves that as humans we are hardwired to move! So we should use the devices on our phones or wrists to motivate us. Take risks and try various forms of exercise till you find what is enjoyable and doable. Start with interval walking (brisk/slow) and gradually make it more challenging as your body learns to integrate and get used to moving again. If you enjoy being social, incorporate activity into time spent with friends or co-workers, join a hiking or biking group, or attend a fitness class. Start slowly and make exercise fun; your health and positive mindset will follow.

Exercise Your Muscles

For most healthy adults, the U.S. Department of Health and Human Services[12] recommends at least 150 minutes per week of moderate aerobic activity[13] or seventy-five minutes per week of vigorous aerobic activity.[14] You can also do a combination of moderate and vigorous activities. Remember, there are three types of exercise and you will want to do two types each day. Even brief bouts of activity offer benefits. For instance, if you can't fit in one thirty-minute walk, try three ten-minute walks instead.

· *Cardio.* Adults need at least thirty to forty-five minutes a day with heart rate over 120 beats per minute. Running, cycling, swimming, and skiing are all great options. Interval training, which entails brief bursts (sixty to ninety seconds) of intense activity at almost full effort, is safe and effective.

· *Strength training.* Our body needs mechanical stress to build strength, and weights are a great way to do this. Start with five pounds and gradually increase to twelve to fifteen pounds. Aim for two sessions a week. Research shows this is enough to preserve bone mass at the spine and hip over two to three years.[15] Remember, this can be as easy as doing push-ups, squats, and other body-weight exercises at home.

· *Stretching.* Adults need daily stretching to improve blood flow, range of motion, and flexibility. You can start with stretching in the shower or before you got to bed. Yoga and Pilates in a structured environment are great ways to integrate the muscles, bones, and fascia to prevent stiffness. The more you "flexercise," the less likely you are to fall.

If you have been inactive, take it easy at first—walk before you run—and then gradually make your workouts more challenging. If you like being outdoors, find an activity you can do in a pleasurable environment. If you want more time with friends, try to enlist them for social activities like dancing or group walks. Your local Y or community health center is a good place to begin. If you are uncomfortable exercising in a health club or other public space, start by working out at home or choose a solo activity like cycling. YouTube has great workouts you can do in the privacy of your own home, including yoga.

Remember, small steps to change your behavior have big outcomes for your lifestyle. Use your mind to embed exercise habits into your brain. Our brain cells need the extra oxygen, blood flow, and growth factors that result from exercise. And our brains become more plastic because new neuronal connections are formed between different areas in the brain. Working out your glutes will directly benefit your gray matter! Exercise also increases serotonin production in the brain, which makes you feel good and improves learning. Exercise is a very effective antidepressant.

$$\longleftrightarrow$$

TRY THESE ADDITIONAL STEPS to develop your movement mindset and make exercise a habit.

➤ Commit to the SMUFLD Formula

Along with the obesity epidemic came a billion-dollar business opportunity... infomercials about gadgets to shrink your belly, increase your thigh muscles, or improve your cardio conditioning. Memberships at gyms and athletic clubs and the hiring of personal trainers have increased. We are paying good money to move. Health research into chronic disease has contributed to this trend, but it doesn't have to be expensive or complicated for us to be active. Use the Smart, Motivation, Urgency, Focus, Leverage, and Decisions (SMUFLD) formula to help you make big changes to your lifestyle, specifically developing a healthier diet and a more active lifestyle.

SMART goals. Setting goals and writing them down is important. SMART stands for *S*pecific, *M*easurable, *A*ttainable, *R*elevant, and *T*ime-limited. If your primary goal is to reduce stress in your life and recharge your batteries, your specific goals might include committing to walking during your lunch hour three times a week. Or if needed, finding a babysitter to watch your children so you can slip away to attend a cycling class.

Motivation. It is important to recognize what drives human behavior. Why do you want to exercise? What do you truly value? Your doctor may want you to lose weight to lower your blood pressure, but if that isn't important to you, the message will not embed into your subconscious. However, if fitness for you means, "I will be able to play soccer with my grandson," that thought may keep you active. Often I use medical markers, such as lowering the cholesterol or blood sugar, to motivate people. While that is helpful, even more effective is figuring out what drives you subconsciously. Instead of asking yourself what is the matter with you, try thinking about what matters to you. What do you love? What do you really want?

Urgency. Urgent matters get priority in the sorting bin of your busy brain. When I give someone a diet plan or exercise suggestions and they say, "I'm going to start this when I retire," or "I'll do this when I get back from vacation," I know that the perfect time will not come. Their subconscious has filed the information for later reference. In contrast, when I hear, "I'm going to start doing this today," I know they have flagged it as a top priority and it will get done. If they repeat this action, it becomes a habit. The instant decision to make changes now is a conscious one. Using your mind to give urgency and priority on a daily basis will help create a permanent, subconscious, and automatic habit for movement.

Focus. While most people complain of lack of time, sometimes it's more a lack of focus. Daily distractions bombard and derail us from what is truly important. How many times do we hear people say, "I had good intentions to go eat a healthy salad . . . but then my friend texted me about a wine-tasting dinner and my diet went out the window"? We always have an excuse for what derailed us. The key to making movement your focus is to zero in on the payoff or goal that allows your brain to hone what's important and then prioritize where you spend your energy. Meditating for just a few minutes in the morning to set your intentions can go a long way to helping with micro decisions throughout the day, because it keeps you more focused on your priorities.

Leverage. What are you willing to give up to reach your goal? You may have to give up a day at the beach so you can write your book (as I'm doing right now). Or give up dessert to lower your blood sugars. Or choose the gym over going for drinks. The key is to reframe what you are giving up, so it feels like honoring what is best for you. Instead of telling yourself, "I hate exercise," perhaps you can try, "I choose to move my body to take care of myself," "I love how I feel after I finish a great workout," or even, "I'm changing my DNA and my health destiny by exercising."

Decisions. Every second of every day, your mind makes micro decisions and communicates with the ANS, which regulates the body's response. Your thoughts create emotions, which result in particular actions or behaviors. You may make a conscious decision to lose weight, but to make this happen, your subconscious mind has to be on board. You have just a few seconds to rewire the brain before it takes over automatically and leads you down a familiar pathway based on past beliefs and ingrained habits. To capture those few seconds before a subconscious automatic pattern takes over, implement the five-second rule.

Mel Robbins uses the principles of neuroscience to set an intention and count backward from five.[16] Many of us have applied the five-second rule when a morsel of food falls to the floor and we proceed to eat it. We rationalize that bacteria are unlikely to grow in five seconds so it must be okay. However, Robbins's five-second rule has to do with how our brain works when we are trying to instill new habits or change our behavior. The rule is simple: you must act on an instinct or desire immediately before your brain kills it. If you hesitate, the five-second window can mean the difference between success and failure for instilling healthier behaviors. Instead of giving in to the familiar and easy path, you choose to act by counting backward: 5-4-3-2-1-go! Counting backward makes you focus on the particular goal or action. Otherwise, you remain stagnant and change will be less likely.

Executive functioning, decision making, planning, and goal setting occur in the prefrontal cortex of the brain. It is known as the "internal locus of control." You can further cultivate this control by pushing past resistance and using "activation energy" to propel you away from familiar, automatic behaviors. Therefore, setting an intention such as "I will go for a walk now" and then counting down from five disrupts the automatic pathway of your body choosing to sit on the couch (familiar, comfortable).

This is one way to push yourself to do hard work that you often avoid, dislike, or are scared to do. The five-second countdown gives you momentum to form a new pathway to new behaviors. Since our body has a "bias toward action," it will act when the brain says to. So when we prune bad habits and establish healthy ones with control and repetition, we will act on them. Use SMUFLD to make exercise your new habit!

Case Study: Judy

Judy prided herself on following a largely plant-based diet and maintaining an ideal weight despite her hectic job as a supervisor at a large telecommunications company. So she was surprised when I informed her that both her blood pressure and her cholesterol levels were high and that she needed to make some lifestyle changes to reduce her risk of heart disease. Judy sat all day long. The obvious solution was to get her to move more.

Judy had led a largely sedentary lifestyle for more than twenty-five years. She understood my concern for her well-being and she wasn't averse to exercise, but she wasn't strongly motivated to get active, until she made the connection that exercise was now the key to maintaining her physical independence in the future. I emphasized to Judy the importance of exercise to relieve stress, reduce heart disease risk, improve brain and immune function, and help build stronger bones. But it was her fear of being dependent on others if she had a stroke or heart attack that drove her to incorporate exercise into her daily routine.

Together we set some SMART goals to help her achieve her health goals:

- Start each day with ten minutes of breath, mind, word (BMW) meditation (page 82) to set a mental intention to be more fit.

- Take two minutes each morning to stretch fully and do a mini BMW meditation in the afternoon to reduce stress and re-set the ANS.

- Walk 5,000 steps every lunch hour (specific, measurable, attainable, and relevant) for ninety days (time-restricted) and then reassess.

Motivation. Once Judy realized that diet was not enough to control her blood pressure and cholesterol levels, adding exercise to stay independent in the future became her primary driving force.

Urgency. She implemented the plan immediately to increase her chance of success.

Focus. Judy wrote down fitness goals and made a plan to do something active every day. She replaced checking work-related emails and texts as a top priority on her daily to-do list with movement and exercise.

Leverage. She had to ease up on always being present, in charge, and important at the office in order to make more time for herself. This trade-off was hard for Judy but also liberating.

Decisions. As Judy became more aware of the risks associated with prolonged sitting, she made a conscious decision to move more. She set an alarm on her phone to remind herself to move or stretch every two hours.

Once Judy established a routine of daily movement, it eventually became an automatic habit. A year after her initial visit, exercise had become a part of her life. Judy's blood pressure and cholesterol were both lower, she had built more muscle, and her risk for heart disease and osteoporosis were also significantly lower.

➤ Do What You Love with People You Enjoy

To make movement a habit, it helps to find activities you really enjoy and do them with people you like. After all, any form of exercise or movement can increase your fitness level and decrease your stress—and being around friends adds to that improved mood. Join an early-morning tai chi class on your way to work. Meet a friend for a lunchtime yoga or spin class. Enlist your co-workers in a "walking" meeting. Make an after-dinner walk a family event. Doing activities with other people has the added benefit of keeping you accountable. When others are waiting for you, you're more likely to get out the door even if you're not motivated. If you enjoy your own company, that's fine too. We all need a break from people sometimes, and it can be a great time to commit to thirty minutes of active gardening bonding with the bees. Or a half-hour swim.

Many people find that being outside feels more natural than going to the gym. And science suggests there's something to that. Walking or riding around lots of trees where the air is rich in oxygen reduces blood pressure, heart rate, and stress hormones. Researchers recommend forest bathing[17] every day. Natural sunlight reaching the retina at the back of our eyes activates hormones that help us to sleep. Exposure to sunlight helps our vitamin D levels as well. When you develop an active routine, it's easy to squeeze in time outside. Take the bus to work and run home. Walk to a local park or green space during your lunch hour. Challenge your co-workers to a game of Frisbee or pickup soccer at break time. Join a corporate dragon-boating team. Ride your bicycle to the grocery store.

What's most important is making regular physical activity an integral part of your lifestyle. If exercise intimidates you and you can't overcome your fears about it, consider counseling or coaching to find strategies to help. And if you haven't exercised for some time and you have health concerns, talk to your doctor before starting a new exercise routine.

➤ Stay Positive and Celebrate Your Successes

Sometimes life happens when you least expect it; a broken ankle, an accident, illness, and even pregnancy can disrupt our exercise routine. But don't sit still for too long. It is important to rest to recover, but try to find other creative ways to stay active (chair yoga, isometric exercises, swimming instead of running). Life is an obstacle course: it's our job to find a way around it, over it, or through it, and we must keep moving. No matter how you choose to move, focus on maintaining a positive movement mindset.

The good news is that we can retrain the muscles in our body to relax, stretch, and flex—even after injury or a period away from exercise. This allows us to increase our range of motion and become mobile once more. There are cases of quadriplegics who couldn't voluntarily move their limbs because of a spinal cord injury reawakening buried muscle memory through very dedicated exercises targeting the specific muscle groups for walking and arm movement. Passively moving and strengthening these muscles helps rewire circuits back to the brain, and some people with spinal cord injuries are able to walk again. Your successes may not be quite so dramatic, but it's important to celebrate them nonetheless, whether your goal is better physical or emotional health.

We can use our body positions and muscles not only to improve our physical health but also to help our mind remember a feeling and signal the brain to change emotions. For example, if you feel nervous, intimidated, and unsure before a job interview, practice standing in a wide stance or power pose.[18] Raise your hands up as if celebrating success. Using a muscular stance makes you feel more powerful and in control. You then show up to the interview in a position of power and control. This is the body-brain-mind connection in action, with the cell-signaling theory at the core. Research proves the brain takes cues from the body, so use that knowledge to develop a healthy movement mindset and take charge of your stress.

The Benefits of Healthy Movement

We all know we should exercise. We list reasons such as being healthy, losing weight, and fighting disease. The question is, Why does exercise bring such profound benefits?

➤ Decreased Stress

One way to get rid of cortisol in the body is to engage in physical activity. Our fight-or-flight reaction creates excessive stress hormones. Since these hormones help us flee to get as far from danger as possible, it makes perfect sense to "run off stress." Initial scientific research has shown that cortisol does temporarily increase during exercise. The key word is "temporarily."

For most people, cortisol rates return to normal following exercise and levels stay lower with regular workouts. One study showed that people who exercised regularly were more adaptable and resilient to the effects of stress. Their body systems became well integrated and could respond efficiently to stress hormones.[19]

➤ Improved Memory

Exercise expands our brain, while stress shrinks it. Exercise promotes the production of neurotransmitters like serotonin, norepinephrine, and gamma-aminobutyric acid (GABA). These chemicals support memory, learning, and mood. They improve our cognitive ability, which is often dulled by stressful events. Many researchers report that exercise improves focus, memory, and concentration. Numerous European schools have adopted exercise breaks in their daily curriculum. Teachers at many centers noticed kids scored consistently better in math when their day was broken up by two or three breaks with even ten to fifteen minutes of exercise each time. Higher performance on cognitive tests is an objective measure.[20] This compels us to incorporate exercise as a mandatory part of an academic curriculum. Exercise makes us smarter!

Physical exercise causes the brain to produce certain proteins such as brain-derived neurotrophic factor (BDNF) in higher quantities. We produce less of this protein as we age, yet it is vital for the growth and repair of brain cells. BDNF is one of the crucial factors in allowing the brain to form new neural pathways (neuroplasticity). Better blood supply to the brain, such as from vigorous exercise, contributes to healthier BDNF levels.

The cognitive effects of BDNF are immense. There are higher levels of BDNF where we store our long-term memory, for example in the hippocampus, which is crucial to learning and retaining new information for a long time. BDNF also controls our hunger signals and can suppress appetite. Research is looking at ways to improve our BDNF for weight control. In summary, when BDNF levels are high we acquire knowledge faster and retain it longer, we are happier, and we maintain a healthier body weight. Exercise is an effective way to raise BDNF to improve all those areas, optimize aging, and reduce stress.

➤ Improved Pain

New imaging techniques have allowed researchers to watch how endorphins interact with the human brain and confirm that they increase after physical activity. These natural painkillers, which are like our own built-in opioids, help to heal and repair the body and can cause a state of euphoria referred to as a "runner's high." There are at least twenty kinds of endorphins, but until now they have been difficult to measure. They are produced by the hypothalamus, pituitary gland, and spinal cord but the receptors they are attracted to are found throughout the brain. That means an overall feeling of euphoria or well-being.

A fast-paced game of tennis, several laps in the pool, sexual activity, a good belly laugh, or dancing can produce the same effect as running when it comes to endorphin release. Meditation, acupuncture, massage therapy, and even breathing deeply also increase your level of endorphins. For people with chronic pain, doing deep breathing exercises increases endorphin production and lowers pain perception.

➤ Improved Mood and Sleep

Exercise improves our mood, energy, and optimism. Regular exercise can increase self-confidence. Furthermore, exercise can relax us, and it can lower the symptoms associated with mild to moderate depression and anxiety. People with chronic depression have low levels of serotonin, but there is evidence to show that serotonin levels increase with physical activity.[21] Exercise also limits the effects of stress chemicals on our brain by reducing circulating levels of cortisol and adrenaline. Exercise reduces inflammation via the immune system; inflammation and depression strongly correlate. Depression often leads to disrupted sleep-wake cycles. Exercise helps to restore the normal circadian rhythm and our sleep-wake cycles so that repair hormones released during sleep can heal the body again (see Reclaim Your Rest, page 209).

The key is that physical activity helps to reduce the daily stress load, tension, and irritations. Think of it as "meditation in motion." Science reveals that doing regular aerobic exercise decreases overall levels of tension, elevates and stabilizes mood, improves sleep, and improves self-esteem. Antianxiety effects occur even after just five minutes of aerobic exercise. Many people who have difficulty sitting to meditate incorporate breath work into their cardio activity such as walking briskly, also called walking meditation.

➤ Reduced Inflammation

Research has already shown that exercise is vitally important for reducing inflammation. The endorphins produced during exercise are an important way to reduce inflammation. Exercise probably helps the liver detoxify and reduces inflammatory markers. And reducing inflammation also benefits the brain, as brain inflammation is associated with dementia and depression.

The Mayo Clinic reports that people who exercise can increase their lifespan by just over seven years.[22] Moderate exercise has abundant effects, such as controlling hypertension and diabetes and preventing Alzheimer's disease. All of these diseases affect brain tissue by causing inflammation. Exercise alone is probably one of the best cures for almost every single chronic disease. Exercise dramatically improves heart health by reducing bad cholesterol (LDL) and increasing good cholesterol (HDL). The best part? Exercise is cheap and effective, and changing a few habits doesn't take too much effort. Light to moderate exercise is simple: take the stairs instead of the elevator or walk the dog for a little longer.

Not only does exercise improve our overall health and longevity, it can also save us a great deal of stress in the short run, since it strengthens our immunity to colds, the flu, and other minor illnesses. In the long run, exercise helps us stay healthier longer and enjoy life more.

CONCLUSION

Movement is vital to our well-being. What began as a means of acquiring food or moving away from danger became an integral component of humans adapting to an ever-changing environment. Exercise has well-known health benefits, including optimal oxygenation of our tissues, removal of toxins from our body, improved cardiac function, and stronger bones. When we are under chronic stress, it is also one of the best ways to expel cortisol from the body. In the past, we underestimated what exercise does for our brain; exercise enhances both mood and memory. We are much more aware that people who exercise create a more resilient body for stress. Vigorous exercise causes all systems to integrate and work well, synchronizing movement and oxygenation so that when physical or emotional stress occurs, the body is better able to cope. Exercise improves sleep and enhances the immune system.

At the core of every individual's psyche lies an inherent drive to move or choose the path of least resistance. The good news is we can cultivate a mindset for exercise by being aware of what drives our automatic behavior and consciously choosing to revise and edit a new program if needed. We can use visualization techniques to imagine, believe, and achieve a healthier and more fit version of ourselves. We can use "activation energy," such as the five-second rule, to take charge of our decisions and launch into healthier habits. And we can use our body's own muscle memory to trigger neural pathways that promote movement. "Use it or lose it" is a valid, science-based phenomenon. Exercise pumps oxygen-rich blood to every cell in the body and helps us to remove toxins from our tissues and organs. It makes the heart beat faster and stronger so it doesn't clog up its own blood vessels. It makes our skeletal muscles become stronger and more elastic so they don't atrophy or fail to support our bony skeleton. Movement keeps us physically and mentally healthy so we can successfully become resilient to stress and adapt to change.

6.

Mind
Your Heart

*The best and most beautiful things in the
world cannot be seen or even touched—
they must be felt with the heart.*
Helen Keller

SELF-ASSESSMENT

While it is well known that genetics, diet, and cholesterol play
a role in heart disease, personality traits and behavior also put
us at a higher risk for heart disease and hypertension. More
evidence is emerging about the important role of stress and
emotions in heart health.

Do you:

· often feel impatient and in a rush?

· feel the need to compete and win all the time?

· easily feel irritated and have a short fuse?

· feel hostile or aggressive?

- focus on achievements and measure your self-worth by them?

- find yourself dominating others?

- often interrupt others?

- clench your jaw or grind your teeth?

- usually feel tense?

- sweat excessively?

- have high blood pressure or an increased heart rate?

Aristotle, along with many other early philosophers and scientists, believed the heart was the center of all human thought, emotion, reason, and consciousness. This would have made sense back then. Intense emotion can often manifest itself as a physical sensation from our heart. The experiences of passion and pain deeply intertwine with an elated or heavy feeling in the chest. Religion, literature, and pop culture further strengthen the belief that the heart is the seat of our soul. For example, the Torah, a holy book of the Jewish faith, describes the death of Isaac's mother from heartbreak after learning Abraham would sacrifice her son. In Shakespeare's *Romeo and Juliet*, Lady Montague dies from grief following Romeo's banishment from the city of Verona. And modern media bombards us with songs, TV shows, and movies that reinforce the idea that our heart dictates our mental and emotional state and influences our physical health.

But modern medicine has come to regard the brain and the mind as the true keys to people's consciousness, memory, emotion, and cognition. And we've therefore come to view the heart as a glorified pump commanded by our brain. This pump is extremely robust, beating over 100,000 times a day to send oxygen-rich blood to miles and miles of blood vessels. However, our heart is not merely a mechanical pump. It has its own cardiac nervous system and can even produce hormones.[1] It has a complex bidirectional flow of information with the brain. In fact, we may have underestimated the many signals traveling from the heart to the brain carrying information about what the heart can sense that may be invisible to the brain.

Usually, the autonomic nervous system (ANS) exerts control over our heart with no conscious input from our mind. It increases our heart rate without thinking, for example when we feel fear or other extreme emotions. By understanding the normal and abnormal responses of the heart, we can cultivate a healthy heart mindset and harness the power of our mind to regulate the heart.

ANATOMY OF A HEALTHY HEART

The heart, blood, and blood vessels make up the cardiovascular system, a word that comes from the Greek *kardia* (heart) and the Latin *vas* (vessel). The human heart contracts an astounding 42 million beats per year, or nearly 3 billion beats in the average lifetime. The heart must pump blood throughout the body every second of every day and night, and it must adjust its speed of delivery according to our activity level. So integral is blood to maintaining life that should blood flow halt, we lose consciousness within seconds. And vital cells within the brain die after only a few minutes without oxygen-rich blood.[2] Thus, heart function is essential to providing the body with the fuel and energy we need to survive.

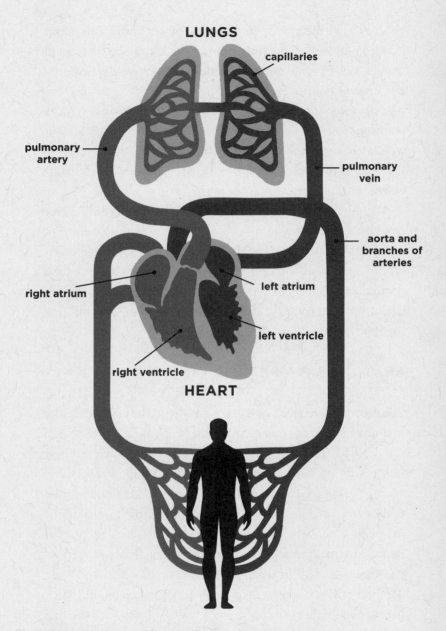

Figure 6.1. A simplified cardiovascular system

Although you can best feel the heartbeat on the left side of the body, the heart actually lies centrally in the chest. This fist-sized organ has four chambers—two atria and two ventricles—composed of specialized muscle tissue (Figure 6.1). The thin-walled atria act as reservoirs for receiving blood. The muscular ventricles provide the pumping power to perfuse our body. Heart muscle, much like the muscle of our arms and legs, squeezes and contracts, pushing the blood of the heart into and out of its connected blood vessels.

One-way valves between the chambers stop blood from moving in the wrong direction, and a muscular wall down the middle separates the right and left sides. The right side of the heart pumps blood to the lungs in a circuit known as pulmonary circulation. The process of pulmonary circulation replenishes the oxygen in the blood while removing the carbon dioxide. The left side of the heart provides systemic circulation, carrying the oxygen-rich blood to the rest of the body. I like to imagine the cardiovascular system as a delivery and pickup service for the body. The delivery hub, or the heart, sends out parcels containing goods needed by its clients. The blood vessels deliver these parcels of oxygen-rich blood to the cells and tissues in the body (clients) and return old boxes to the hub where they become waste.

Pause for a moment to feel your own heart beating. Most people will feel a rhythmic pulsation just below their left nipple. This is your left ventricle pushing against your chest wall, working as hard as it does each and every day. Does it feel fast? Does it feel slow? Do you notice anything different? Being aware of your heart and heart rate is a step toward noticing the connection of your emotional state to the ANS.

The Heart as a Transportation Network:
Arteries, Veins, and Capillaries

The blood vessels are the transportation network allowing parcels to be delivered and collected. Delivery occurs first under high pressure along large highways—the arteries—and then along smaller residential streets—the capillaries. After reaching the customer, collection is the process of returning blood to the heart through a separate network—the veins.

The systemic circulation of oxygenated blood begins with the left ventricle supplying large arteries, such as the aorta. These arteries divide into progressively smaller branches until they are a fraction of the thickness of a human hair. These capillaries are so small that red blood cells, the tiny oxygen-carrying parcels, have to travel in single file. The capillaries are the sites of gas and nutrient exchange between the blood cells and the surrounding tissues and organs.

At the farthest end of the capillaries, the parcel service initiates a return. These veins increase in size as they move away from the client. Larger and larger veins join to form massive vessels, similar to the aorta, which return blood to the right side of the heart. These veins contain used packages that have blood with low oxygen and high carbon dioxide, which must be recycled. From the right atrium and ventricle, blood flows to the lungs where it is replenished with oxygen and the carbon dioxide is exhaled.

Though it may seem odd at first, the heart muscle cannot absorb oxygen from the blood being pumped through it. Like other organs, it needs its own blood vessels! These vessels, called the coronary arteries, branch off from the aorta and carry oxygen-rich blood to supply the powerful heart muscle.

To use our traffic analogy, backup in the hub, traffic on the roads, and problems with the parcels can all cause breakdown of the delivery service. Respectively, changes to the heart, blood vessels, and blood affect the cardiovascular system. When the coronary arteries become blocked by plaque buildup or a blood clot, the blockage disrupts the blood flow to the heart muscle, causing it to malfunction and stop pumping blood—a heart attack.

The Heart as a Communication Network: Electrical, Neurological, and Biochemical Pathways

How does our mind enter the picture? Electrical cells within the walls of our heart stimulate the contractions, or what we know as the heartbeat. These electrical signals spread throughout the muscle, causing the heart to squeeze and push blood out. The electrical cells, known collectively as the sinoatrial node, form the pacemaker within the heart and induce contraction without any input from the brain. Pacemaking cells are self-sustaining and give a natural heart rate of 60 to 100 beats per minute in adults.

However, the pacemaker does not act alone. Nerves stretching from the brain and brainstem connect extensively around the heart and into the sinoatrial node (Figure 6.2). By collecting information about a situation, the brain determines the optimal heart rate for each moment and circumstance. This clever system uses an unconscious series of checks and balances to constantly tweak our cardiac output. Specialized receptors in the neck detect our blood pressure, oxygenation, and the amount of carbon dioxide in the blood. For example, during vigorous exercise, the working muscles consume much of the oxygen in the blood, causing our oxygen level to drop. The cardiovascular receptors detect this physical demand and deficit in oxygen. Within seconds, signals pass through sympathetic nerves to kick-start the system, increasing our heart rate and our breathing rate to ensure the muscles receive the oxygen they need.

Unfortunately, this clever system also has a fatal flaw. We know our body reacts to external information (for example, exercise) and can change our heart rate. However, our mind may also affect the heart, responding to internal stimuli. Fear, stress, anxiety, and other emotions can act on this system. In the few instances I have watched horror movies, my heart fluttered rapidly in my chest while I gripped the arms of my chair. You can probably think of a time when your own heart rate increased without any physical demand.

The increase in heart rate is part of our fight-or-flight reaction due to stress. Our subconscious mind uses the sympathetic nervous system (SNS) to arouse our organ systems during stressful circumstances, which can range from running a marathon to starting the first day of school. In the cardiovascular system, our SNS conducts sensory and motor functions. Think of sensory functions as similar to our senses of taste, hearing, and touch, where nerves from our tongue, ears, and skin travel to our brain. Here, the nerves are going from our heart to our brain and detect increases or decreases in blood pressure and gas levels.

During a stressful event, the sympathetic nerves are activated. Neural connections from the brainstem to our heart increase signal rates and the force of contractions, while nerves to blood vessels cause constriction to increase our blood pressure.

Under physical circumstances, these stress-induced changes are not harmful and are in fact crucial in life-or-death situations.

BRAIN

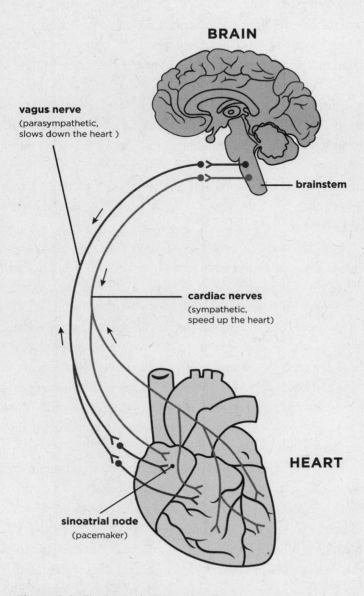

vagus nerve
(parasympathetic,
slows down the heart)

brainstem

cardiac nerves
(sympathetic,
speed up the heart)

HEART

sinoatrial node
(pacemaker)

Figure 6.2. The heart–brain connection

For example, if you are in a car accident and undergo major blood loss, your fight-or-flight reaction kicks into action. It will divert blood from the site of injury toward vital organs like the heart and brain to minimize blood loss and keep you alive. However, long-term activation of the stress response from internal stimuli may cause a wide variety of diseases, such as hypertension (prolonged constriction of blood vessels). For our heart health, we need to understand that the stressed mind increases signals going to the adrenal gland, which surges out cortisol and adrenaline. These chemicals increase our risk for heart attack and stroke and make us more prone to heart attacks when acute distress occurs.

Our counterpart to the SNS (gas) is of course the parasympathetic nervous system (PNS; brakes). This relaxing drive lets the brain communicate with the heart via the vagus nerve. Its influence slows heart rate and the force of contractions. The vagus nerve loosens tightness in the chest and is responsible for feelings of calm throughout the body. A strong balance exists between SNS and PNS in healthy individuals. The PNS should only hand over control to the SNS to pump up the heart during times of true physical demand. Recognizing the difference between the two allows us to exert control over our own autonomic nervous system.

In modern times, we are learning how our internal mental dialogue can create visceral responses even when an external input is absent. That is, our heart rate can vary without the brain telling it to. The new field of neurocardiology shows that the heart muscle has a complex system of powerful neural pathways that behave independently, and our heart rate is under the control of different systems, including the ANS. Neurotransmitter proteins, peptides (tiny proteins), and hormones that behave like the ones in the brain contribute to the dynamic state of the heart. We need the constant dialogue between the heart and the brain so we can adjust our heartbeat to our external environment. I believe I can teach you how to adjust your heartbeat for your internal environment. Therefore, understanding the deep connection between our emotional state and our heart is essential.

When overburdened by constant emotional stress, excessive physical effort, and lack of proper rest, the heart becomes vulnerable to disease. In extreme cases, people have dropped dead in their office due to heart failure brought on by overwork. This phenomenon, known as *karoshi* in Japanese, literally means "overwork death." In one example, Miwa Sado accumulated a whopping 159 hours of overtime in July 2013 before she died while working for a prominent Japanese broadcaster in Tokyo.[3] That's *nineteen standard workdays* on top of her regular schedule. Although I'm not aware of any postmortem studies of her heart, I believe stress-related heart failure played a significant part in her death.

More research has investigated silent or sudden cardiac deaths that occur in North America in stressed individuals, and results support the role of stress hormones in heart disease. Cushing's syndrome is a condition in which the body produces too much cortisol. This hormone is usually produced by too much stress, but with Cushing's syndrome it can be caused by a tumor on the adrenal or pituitary gland or by overuse of steroid medication. The result is that patients develop wide purple stretch marks as fat accrues in the face, neck, and abdomen. Insulin resistance, diabetes, atherosclerosis, and hypertension accompany these outward changes. And even when people with Cushing's syndrome are treated, they often die prematurely from forms of cardiovascular disease: heart attacks, strokes, and arrhythmias.[4]

We know chronic stress is linked to the severity and prognosis of these conditions. Negative emotions such as anxiety, frustration, lack of control, anger, irritation, and resentment gradually create an imbalance both in the mind and in the nervous system of the heart. It is important to note here that emotions differ from thoughts. For example, just thinking about a heated argument may not create an increased heart rate. However, attaching the emotion of anger to the argument memory re-creates the same visceral response of increased heart rate as being in the argument.

UNDERSTANDING STRESS HORMONES AND OUR HEART

In the world of cardiology, we have been busy trying to treat hypertension and high cholesterol to prevent people from developing heart disease. While these are extremely important interventions, perhaps we have not put enough emphasis on mental health as another root cause of heart disease. A pioneering and popular scientific study in the field of emotions and their effects on heart disease was done in the 1950s, when cardiologists Meyer Friedman and Ray Rosenman looked at the effects of personality type on coronary artery disease by comparing people with type A and type B personalities.[5]

People with a type A personality are characterized as organized, ambitious, outgoing, proactive, and competitive. They are especially aware of time constraints and are always running on all cylinders in every aspect of their life. People with a type A personality often experience high stress. In contrast, people with a type B personality are said to maintain a slower-paced life, take a more patient and relaxed approach to situations, and may be more introverted. Type B people have less intrinsic drive to achieve and conquer, and they experience less stress. Obviously, more than two personality types exist and the authors were criticized for this oversimplification when they published the results of their study. Nonetheless, their conclusions provide insight into how stress affects our heart health.

Published in 1959 in the *Journal of the American Medical Association*, this study was one of the first to investigate how changes in the mind can affect the body. The researchers grouped nearly 200 men according to their personality type and behavior patterns and then followed them for over eight years. At the end of the study, the researchers concluded that individuals with a type A personality were twice as likely to develop heart disease, even after they controlled for lifestyle factors such as smoking and alcohol use. Several further studies over the past half-century have corroborated this fact: our state of mind affects our heart health.[6] In my own practice, I have seen that by exposing ourselves to consistently high levels of stress, we expose ourselves to the risk of heart disease.

Chronic stress, poor adaptability, or low resilience to stress creates a negative emotional footprint, which is the backdrop of depression and anxiety. If you suffer from one of these mental conditions, the other likely affects you as well. The latest medical research has added a third condition. Over the past decade, researchers have been linking the statistics and noticing that depression accelerates heart disease. Scientists at the Johns Hopkins University School of Medicine studied over 1,000 male medical students and determined that those who scored highest on depression inventory scales had a twofold increase in the likelihood of developing heart disease.[7] The more severe the depression, the greater the risk for heart disease. While depression is an independent factor, the study also showed that people diagnosed with a heart condition were more likely to have depression and anxiety as an emotional response to heart disease itself. A diagnosis of a life-threatening illness is a huge stressor to the mind and creates fear, and we know survivors of heart attacks in North America often experience a major depression after the attack. Not only have they faced possible death, but they also have to make profound adjustments to their lives. Failure to adapt to those new changes puts them in a higher risk category, adding to their stress.

How Stress Affects Our Heart

Our heart health is vital to life itself. When our heart isn't working properly, it compromises blood flow and oxygen supply to every tissue in the body, including the heart muscle. Whether due to our personality type or our lifestyle, our state of mind can have an impact on our heart.

Stress hormones can play a large role in heart problems. As we've seen, chronic stress causes excessive levels of circulating cortisol and adrenaline, which directly affect the function of the heart muscle, such as electrical conduction in the heart or spasm in the coronary vessels. These hormones cause blood vessels to constrict and thereby increase the rate of the resting heartbeat and blood pressure. We know adrenaline stimulates the heart since it is directly injected into the heart muscle when trying to revive a person in cardiac arrest. However, cortisol and adrenaline can also indirectly damage the heart. Several heart conditions are directly related to stress.

➤ Hypertension

Hypertension is another word to describe high blood pressure. The Centers for Disease Control and Prevention states that one in three adult Americans has high blood pressure.[8] Known as the "silent killer," it is an especially dangerous condition because though it can be fatal, it has nearly no symptoms. A person with high blood pressure may never know of their condition unless a doctor diagnoses it or they collapse. The lack of specific symptoms also makes it difficult to treat: many patients stop taking their antihypertensive drugs because they develop side effects, not realizing that the medications were working to reduce their unseen symptoms.

Our arteries can adapt to high pressure for short periods of time—the muscular walls allow a great range of blood pressures to occur while still maintaining blood flow. But chronic stress means that hormone levels don't drop off as they should, arterial muscles stay constricted longer, and they sustain damage. Cortisol and adrenaline, the hormones associated with stress, strain our blood vessels in this way. When our arteries have been under constant strain for many years, the walls lose their elasticity and become more constricted, decreasing blood supply to the skin and vital organs. As a result, hypertension is the leading risk factor for heart attacks and strokes. Reducing stress has been shown to reduce blood pressure.

Case Study: Abdul

Abdul had been my patient for a few years and had presented with high blood pressure on several visits, likely because of his family history, weight, shift work, poor diet, and lack of exercise. He was in his late fifties and drove a taxi six nights a week to support his wife, son, and daughter. During one visit, his blood pressure readings were especially high and I took the opportunity to investigate further.

He complained of some shortness of breath and so I referred him to a cardiologist for stress testing. He was placed on several medications: beta-blockers to lower his blood pressure, statins to bring down his cholesterol, and a diuretic to get rid of extra fluid in his body. I knew from his lifestyle and the timing of his symptoms that stress played a role, and I initially gave him some information on diet and exercise. I also helped to treat the side effects from the drugs: the dizziness and impotence from his beta-blocker, the muscle fatigue from his statins, and the loss of too much potassium caused by his diuretic.

Abdul was unhappy. His hypertension had given him no symptoms, yet the blood pressure drugs were causing unpleasant side effects. I realized I needed to understand and treat the root cause of the sudden rise in his blood pressure. As we talked, I discovered that Abdul had worked as an electrical engineer in his home country of Lebanon. In North America, his engineering skills were not recognized and so he drove a cab. His culture expected that he would support his wife, mentor his son, and protect his daughter—all while providing the best life for his family. In reality, they were living hand to mouth. His wife was battling depression and his son was hanging around with a rough group of friends—drinking and smoking almost every evening. To top it off, he had just found out that his daughter was dating a man of a different faith. To escape his problems, Abdul spent much of his free time eating junk food and watching TV. It was clear that he was living in a constant state of fight-or-flight reaction and that his cortisol and adrenaline levels were likely high.

Though we could not immediately change his stressors, we could address his response to them. I explained the mind-brain-body connection and walked him through the breath, mind, word (BMW) relaxation techniques (page 82). I also referred him for counseling so he could learn to see past his circumstances and frame a healthier perspective. After a few months of counseling and practicing the BMW stress-reduction techniques, he started exercising and eating properly. He was sleeping better too! We were able to reduce his medications to just one prescription for fluid retention to use as needed. His energy and outlook improved remarkably, though he still had occasional high blood pressure readings when stress and late-night shifts got the best of him. Most importantly, Abdul felt empowered by knowing he could regulate his own response to the stressors and keep his blood pressure in check naturally.

➤ Heart Attack

A heart attack, or more technically myocardial infarction, is one of the most common causes of mortality in our society. The prefix "myo" refers to muscle and "cardial" to the heart, and an infarction occurs when the blood supply is cut off from an area of tissue. Thus, a heart attack describes an obstruction of blood flow—a buildup of plaque or a blood clot (or both)—to the pumping heart muscle. Once the heart loses oxygen and nutrient supply, it ceases to function. And that failing or failed pump can't supply the brain or other vital organs, quickly leading to death.

Chronic stress increases our risk of heart attack because it creates inflammation in the body by desensitizing the immune system to cortisol. Furthermore, stress hormones can cause our coronary arteries to go into spasm even when there is no blockage. For example, young people using cocaine but with no other risk factors for a heart attack frequently present with constricted coronary arteries in spasm that can lead to deadly heart rhythms. The drug kicks hormones and the SNS into overdrive, which leads to the "high" feelings of increased energy and overheating, but this sudden rush of stimulation can also lead to heart attack.

Many medical, familial, and lifestyle factors can increase our risk of suffering a heart attack. For example, hypertension, high cholesterol, and diabetes can damage blood vessels throughout the body, including the coronary arteries that supply the heart. Genetics play an important role because diseases affecting the heart can run in families, but our DNA is not necessarily our destiny. Drinking, smoking, eating poorly, being sedentary, and experiencing sleep deprivation—all frequent side effects of stress—increase the risk of heart attack. Fear, anger, hostility, and distress are also common emotional contributors.

On January 17, 1994, an earthquake measuring 6.7 on the Richter scale struck the Los Angeles area. It jolted millions of people awake at 4:31 a.m. as their houses shook and shuddered. Nearly sixty people died as a direct cause of the earthquake, and approximately 10,000 people were injured. A few clever researchers recognized this tragic event as a unique opportunity to see how this sudden emotional and psychological strain affected people's hearts. Not included in the death toll was a 500 percent increase in sudden cardiac death on the day of the earthquake. In the week preceding the disaster, a daily average of 4.6 people died suddenly from heart attacks. However, on January 17, a whopping twenty-four people died from the same cause.[9]

This stunning story really shows the power of our emotional state on our heart. The acute distress caused by the earthquake triggered heart attacks in up to two dozen people. They may already have had a higher chance of a heart attack from chronic stress or poor lifestyle creating background inflammation, and all it took was an acute stressor, such as that earthquake, to put them over the limit.

Case Study: Jason

Jason was an oil executive based out of Houston, Texas, who shouldered a lot of financial responsibility for international drilling sites and was in charge of high-level employee contracts. He traveled extensively for work, ate out frequently, and had no time to exercise. Although he'd had occasional high blood pressure readings in middle age, he had no evidence of established coronary heart disease.

With the economic downturn, the oil companies were losing a lot of money and Jason's supervisor had asked him to let 150 employees go without notice. Many of these people had become loyal friends and colleagues over three decades of working together, and Jason felt very uncomfortable about delivering the bad news. His chest felt heavy. Just before the big meeting at which Jason was to announce the layoffs, he suffered a sudden and unexpected major heart attack.

Jason's heart attack was like a perfect storm: his life-style of chronic stress had been slowly building toward cardiac arrest, and I believe the swift surge of stress hormones from having to lay off his employees was the triggering event. Literally and figuratively, he did not have the heart to let so many people go. Fortunately, Jason reached the hospital in time and had cardiac intervention with angioplasty and a stent. He has since recovered and taken a less-stressful job, and more importantly, he has cultivated a new mindset around heart health.

➤ Stroke

A stroke is like a heart attack in the brain. A blood clot or ruptured blood vessel prevents blood flow from reaching brain tissue, resulting in damage to the tissue or death. Brain cells can die at a shocking rate of 1.9 million per minute without oxygen,[10] which makes stroke the fifth-highest cause of death and a major cause of disability in the United States.[11] But what does stroke have to do with the heart and stress?

The prolonged exposure to stress hormones that causes blood vessels to constrict can result in high blood pressure that damages the walls of the blood vessels in the brain as well as in the atria of the heart. Cortisol and adrenaline both promote chemicals of inflammation and activate platelets that promote clotting in blood vessels of the heart and the brain. Blood clots that form in the heart often go directly to the brain.

➤ Arrhythmia

The heart has a normal rhythm with a specific electrical pattern that can be measured on an electrocardiogram (EKG). Sometimes an abnormal rhythm—a flutter or a brief pause known as an arrhythmia—occurs. Some arrhythmias have no symptoms but others can make you feel dizzy or faint. Some cause the heart to slow down too much, called *bradycardia*, and others cause a high heart rate, called *tachycardia*. Negative emotions such as stress, anger, and depression have a significant effect on heart rhythm and rate. Stress hormones contribute to narrowing blood vessels and increasing inflammation markers, and they impair certain blood cells like platelets. We now know stress also affects the natural "pacemakers" of our heart.

The story, however, does not end with the heart. The signals from the heart go back to the brain and have an impact on regions of the brain, creating physical changes we can measure on an MRI. Some people seem to be more susceptible than others. Why? The ANS plays a critical role in regulating the heart-brain pathways and may determine how a person learns to respond from both a heart rate and a behavior standpoint. Stress and anger are associated with surges in circulating adrenaline, which stimulates the heart to beat faster. While the heart muscle can withstand short bursts of adrenaline intermittently, exposure to constant high levels of adrenaline is harmful. Chronic stress increases both the frequency of arrhythmia and the chance of death.

➤ My Story

During my lifetime, I have generally had a resting heart rate of 56 to 60 beats per minute. (You can count your pulse for fifteen seconds and multiply it by four to get your resting heart rate.) Following my car accident, I experienced occasional "flutters" when I felt excruciating pain or if I woke up with a nightmare about the accident. After some time, I noticed my resting heart rate had increased even when I was not in pain or when I was feeling relaxed. My resting heart rate shifted to 72 to 80 beats per minute, which is still within the normal range but was higher than my normal.

On one particularly stressful day, I woke with a lot of pain after a terrible night of insomnia and felt the "flutters" in my heart. Later, I received news that my first cousin had died in a car accident. I was shocked and devastated; he was my age and we were very close. For the rest of the day, I could feel my heart racing and I felt dizzy and breathless. I checked my heart rate, and it was well over 120. My husband insisted we go to the emergency department that evening. The EKG registered my heart at 170 beats per minute. A cardiologist conducted various tests and determined that the combination of chronic and acute stress and a viral infection of my thyroid had contributed to the sudden and dangerous rise in heart rate. Very high levels of thyroid hormone can dramatically increase the heart rate. To slow down my heart rate, he prescribed beta-blockers, which I had to take for several weeks until it settled.

➤ Takotsubo Cardiomyopathy

In rare critical cases, severe emotional stress—a bad romantic breakup or the death of a loved one—can send a huge surge of stress hormones through the body that causes the heart to balloon. This condition is known as takotsubo cardiomyopathy (from the Japanese word *takotsubo*, "octopus trap," which describes the round shape of a ballooned heart), or more commonly stress cardiomyopathy or "broken heart" syndrome.[12] The unusually large surge of adrenaline and cortisol puts a huge strain on the left ventricle. Small vessels within the heart tighten and close, starving the organ of oxygen, which cause the muscular ventricular walls to expand outward in a process known as "ballooning." Patients with this condition experience chest pain and shortness of breath, and doctors often believe their patients are having a heart attack. Luckily, X-rays and ultrasound clearly show the swollen apex of the heart and most patients survive the initial event. Their heart muscle returns to its original shape, and they recover physically within a few weeks. In other words, a "broken heart" is not literally a destroyed heart. However, it is another very tangible example of the profound mind-body connection.

HOW TO CULTIVATE
A HEALTHY HEART MINDSET

Stress can start, speed up, or worsen heart disease and there is a direct correlation between stress load and cardiac function. Although stress is an inevitable part of life, some of us are naturally more adaptable and resilient than others. Yet, we can learn to cultivate a healthy heart mindset. For example, we know that depression can cause and complicate heart disease, and over

80 percent of patients diagnosed with depression can successfully be treated by psychotherapy, meditation, and/or counseling. Can antidepressants treat heart disease? It would appear so, but more research is needed. Some specialty clinics are adding medication to treat depression following heart attacks. In contrast, we can say with certainty that a stress management program reduces the chances that a heart patient will need surgery and can be very important to help prevent heart disease.

A number of studies have demonstrated the effectiveness of stress management therapy. In a study of both men and women, patients receiving stress management therapy had lower rates of cardiac events than those receiving only traditional cardiac rehabilitation.[13] The authors suggest that stress management should be routinely incorporated into cardiac rehabilitation programs. Similarly, a Swedish study found that stress reduction prolongs life in women with coronary disease, with an almost three-fold protective effect of the intervention.[14]

By learning to regulate our ANS to meet the challenges of everyday stressors, we create neural pathways that encourage the heart to produce chemicals that improve circulation and work as anti-inflammatory agents, and we cause the mind to allow emotions and behaviors that align with sustainable health. So how do we do this? In addition to meditation and deep breathing techniques, which are very effective, here are some other methods to optimize heart health.

Regulate Your Heart Rate
Biofeedback is the technique of recording the body's involuntary processes, such as heart rate and brain waves, in order to learn how to control them. It is based on the science that emotions affect the ANS, and these can be measured as changes

in electrical patterns, skin conductance, blood pressure, and hormone levels. The underlying premise is that our emotions move faster than our thoughts, and the heart's nervous system registers them before the brain. The heart pulses out an electrical rhythm that is transmitted to the brain, which then registers the signal. By attaching sensors to a patient and recording these wave patterns, we can learn to recognize disordered thinking and deliberately change our mindset.

The HeartMath Institute[15] carries out research and uses biofeedback to help patients reduce stress using meditation and deep breathing techniques. In their labs, patients are hooked up to an electroencephalogram (EEG) and/or an electrocardiogram (EKG) that measure the electrical patterns of the brain and heart, respectively. Anxiety, for example, shows up as slightly chaotic brain waves. By teaching patients to meditate, breathe deeply, and visualize calm and positive images, clinicians can help them relax and achieve a coherent pattern between the heart and the brain. The heart mirrors precisely what is happening in the brain. HeartMath is a great tool that merges biology with technology to help teach your body self-regulation. Over time, patients learn to control their heart and brain-wave patterns so they can produce hormones that promote health and well-being, not stress.

←——→

TRY THESE ADDITIONAL STEPS to regulate your heart rate.

➤ Quit Smoking
Smoking, whether daily or just occasionally, is a major risk factor for heart disease because the chemicals in tobacco smoke harm blood cells and damage the heart and blood vessels. Plaque accumulates more readily in damaged arteries and

veins, reducing the flow of oxygenated blood to the organs and other parts of the body. When combined with other risk factors—such as high cholesterol, high blood pressure, and overweight or obesity—smoking further raises the risk of heart disease. If you smoke, ask your doctor for help quitting.

The most effective programs frame smoking within the context of a patient's life and begin by addressing barriers to quitting. Upgrading your inner dialogue (page 28) is very helpful as a starting point here. Ask yourself, Which cigarette do I most look forward to? Which cigarette will be the hardest to give up? When will I feel most challenged during my attempt to quit? How ready do I feel to make this change? When you can answer these questions, you can tap into your conscious brain (page 55). Smoking-cessation programs then further arm quitters with the tools—education, counseling, and pharmaceutical support—to be successful.

➤ Choose a Heart-Healthy Diet

We know our heart is intimately connected to our mind and brain. To take care of our heart means increasing our overall health, and lifestyle factors play a big role. To protect your heart, limit your intake of processed foods, including sugar, flour, salt, and smoked meats. These ingredients increase your risk of developing hypertension and diabetes, and smoked and cured meats contain cancer-causing nitrates.

A heart-healthy diet should be largely plant-based and high in fiber, omega-3 fatty acids, natural clean fats, and clean proteins. That is, the meat, dairy, and protein sources are grass-fed, free range, and free of antibiotics and steroids. Fresh wild salmon and seafood are staples. I include lots of nuts, seeds, and great oils and fats, including extra-virgin olive oil for salads and unheated foods and grapeseed oil or coconut oil for high-temperature cooking and roasting. I add loads of berries when in season and keep the calorie-rich fruits to a minimum. I also keep refined carbs (sugar and white flour) to an absolute minimum. Ultimately, the exact foods you eat are up to you—just aim for a heart-healthy diet that you can follow at least 90 percent of the time. And if food sensitivities are a problem for you, consider using the 5R gut program (page 110).

In addition to cleaning up your food choices, reduce your alcohol intake to less than one drink per day, and avoid episodes of binge drinking. Consume caffeine in limited quantities (one to two cups), especially if your heart rate increases following a cup of coffee. Getting your blood pressure and blood sugar levels checked regularly is also a heart-healthy precaution.

➤ Make Regular Exercise a Priority

We know that thirty minutes of regular cardio exercise moves oxygen-rich blood to the heart to help grow new cells and repair and heal damaged ones. Furthermore, regular movement builds the heart's resilience, which helps stave off heart disease and promotes healthy aging. Exercise also helps you maintain a healthy weight and avoid conditions such as high blood pressure, high cholesterol, and type 2 diabetes, which can lead to heart disease. See Exercise Your Muscles (page 143).

➤ Aim for Seven to Nine Hours of Quality Sleep
  Every Night

A lack of quality sleep makes it difficult to maintain a health mindset. When we are physically and mentally exhausted all the time, we tend to make poor choices around diet, exercise, and other lifestyle factors. These lead to increased stress, which raises blood pressure, reduces our mood, and is associated with higher risks of obesity and heart disease. See Reclaim Your Rest (page 209).

The Benefits of a Healthy Heart

Cardiovascular disease is the leading cause of death among men and women in the United States and, in fact, worldwide. In 2017, heart-related conditions accounted for slightly less than a quarter (23.5%) of all deaths in the United States.[16] For this reason alone, maintaining a healthy heart is one of the best ways of increasing our life expectancy. After all, a trained and healthy heart works more efficiently and beats at a lower rate when the body is resting, which means that it works less over time and does not wear out.

A healthy heart allows us to be more active, and that consistent movement is associated with greater happiness, healthy body weight, and lower incidence of lifestyle diseases such as obesity, type 2 diabetes, and certain types of cancer. Better physical health leads to greater emotional and mental health, so keep your heart healthy, and your brain and body will follow!

CONCLUSION

The root cause of heart disease is a combination of genetics, medical history, and lifestyle factors. Integrative medicine also shows us the powerful links between emotional attitudes and physiological well-being and longevity. In other words, our heart and brain are collecting information and communicating with each other at all times and affecting our health.

All of us cope with fears of death, illness, loneliness, rejection, and failure. If we don't calm our minds, these fears signal

the brain to produce adrenaline and cortisol and we experience
a stress reaction. When these emotional reactions occur daily,
they become automatic. They can become so habitual that they
actually form part of our personality. It is therefore not enough
to treat heart patients with medication; we must also address
their state of mind. Practice mindfulness and relaxation breathing to slow down the heart, improve circulation, and lower blood
pressure. Improved cardiac outcomes and true heart health are
possible only when we cultivate a healthy heart mindset. Keep
calm so your heart can carry on.

7.

Mind Your Sleep

Sleep is that golden chain that ties health and our bodies together.
Thomas Dekker

SELF-ASSESSMENT

Sleep is vital to our health and well-being. People who don't sleep well are less focused and less productive. They often suffer from various ailments and get sick. People have taken desperate measures for a good night's sleep. Take this sleep assessment to gauge your own sleep mindset.

Do you:

- feel anxious about going to bed?

- have trouble falling asleep at night?

- wake in the middle of the night and have difficulty going back to sleep?

- have an erratic sleep schedule?

- snore excessively or stop breathing at night?

- wake up only to an alarm?

- drink two or more cups of coffee during the day to stay awake?

- consume more than two to four alcoholic beverages a day?

- deal with unexplained weight gain around the middle?

- take medications for conditions such as sinus congestion?

- have a habit of checking the phone and emails before going to bed?

Being sleep-deprived seems like a badge of honor in North America, where some companies expect employees to rack up eighty-plus-hour workweeks. Plus, it seems to be the norm for ambitious, high-achieving business grads who equate getting ahead with a lack of sleep. This mindset also spills over to shift workers and other people in high-pressure jobs.

In the medical world, interns and residents used to work a thirty-six-hour shift every third night followed by two eight-hour days. But even residency programs have now shortened the thirty-six-hour shifts to a maximum of twenty-four hours, because they've realized that physician fatigue sometimes resulted in medical errors. Long shifts and disordered sleep are common for many physicians and medical students. Senior doctors justify these as par for the course: the price students pay to get to higher positions.

A chronic lack of sleep, however, is not getting any of us ahead. Instead, disrupted sleep is making us sick, depressed, and unfocused. It is making us fat and accelerating the aging process. While normal sleep heals and repairs the body to keep us in optimal health, disrupted sleep negatively affects the body in many ways. Disrupted sleep has a strong correlation with chronic stress and anxiety, is associated with chronic diseases, and is strongly linked to mood disorders and increased risk for dementia. The good news is that by understanding what healthy sleep is and the effective tools to achieve it, we can create a solid foundation to restore energy, vitality, mood, and memory.

SLEEP 101: NORMAL SLEEP CYCLES

The human body has a natural sleep-wake cycle. For most of us, six to eight hours of sleep (at night) and sixteen to eighteen hours of being awake during daylight are ideal. This daily pattern that naturally determines when it's time to sleep and when it's time to be awake is called the circadian rhythm (Figure 7.1). Circadian rhythm is largely regulated by daylight, hormones, mealtimes, activity level, and the presence or absence of stressors. It is like a built-in clock that helps our cells, glands, and tissues to function properly and it requires little calibration from us. These biological rhythms are not unique to humans; most animals and plants have them as well. Historically, species that had the ability to predict what their environment was going to be like were ultimately more successful than those that could not.

Physically, the circadian clock is located in the suprachiasmatic nucleus (SCN) in the hypothalamus of the brain. There are actually two SCNs, one in each hemisphere of the brain, each containing 20,000 neurons in an area the size of a pinhead. The individual neurons follow a rhythm of activity that ranges between 23.5 and 24.5 hours, but they fall into perfect synchronicity when they work together.

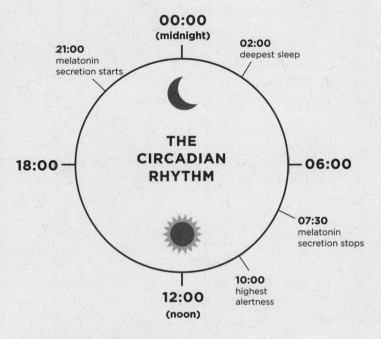

Figure 7.1. The circadian rhythm

To make sure our body clock stays accurate and on schedule each day, the SCN relies on a number of external cues (Figure 7.2). When exposed to light, special light-sensitive cells in the retina of the eye stimulate the optic nerve, which alerts the SCN. The light-dark cycle (day and night), as well as temperature and meal timing, also helps to prevent small timing errors from accumulating and causing serious imbalance in the circadian rhythm. Secondary body clocks in organs such as the heart, the lungs, and the intestines are also influenced by and provide independent feedback to the SCN about timing. By the time we are about six months old, we have more or less developed our regular sleep-wake cycle. And although "morning people" and "night owls" may get up earlier or go to bed later than the average, they typically vary no more than two hours from "normal."

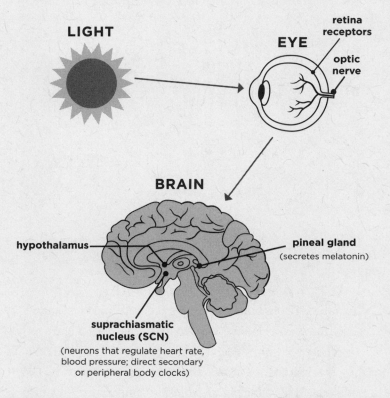

Figure 7.2. How external factors cue the body's circadian rhythm

The SCN sends signals to several other parts of the brain to regulate the body's daily sleep-wake cycle, its temperature, and its hormone production. For example, we know that melatonin, a hormone produced by the pineal gland that causes drowsiness and lowers body temperature, rises as it gets dark in the late afternoon and evening. This is the signal for sleep. In the early morning, melatonin drops. This is one of the signals for wakefulness. Other hormones such as cortisol, prolactin, and thyroid and growth hormones are also involved to signal body arousal.

Circadian rhythms on their own are not enough to cause and regulate sleep. We also have an internal system called the sleep-wake homeostasis that reminds the body it needs to sleep after a certain time. The longer we have been awake, the stronger the desire and need to sleep becomes, and the more likely we are to fall asleep. In contrast, the longer we have been asleep, the more the pressure to sleep disappears, and the more likely we are to wake up. Throughout the day, the SCN sends out alert pulses to the cerebral cortex to keep us aroused and to counteract feelings of drowsiness. In the late evening, however, the circadian rhythm slacks off its alerting system and begins to produce melatonin instead. We don't understand exactly how this shift happens, but as long as the drive for sleep is stronger than the drive for arousal, the body will wind down and prepare for sleep.

Sleep is a time for physical rest. It is also the time when the body heals and repairs tissues. For example, during sleep the pituitary gland releases growth hormone essential to tissue repair. It also produces the hormone prolactin, which helps to regulate metabolism, lactation, and immunity. Oxytocin, a hormone produced in the hypothalamus and associated with childbirth, reaches its peak in the body after five hours of sleep and supports our emotional well-being, social behavior, and dreaming. The brain even produces a hormone that allows us to sleep through the night without the need to urinate. Proper sleep regulates the normal functioning of these chemicals and hormones, as well as others such as dehydroepiandrosterone (DHEA), a hormone associated with our health and longevity.

Sleep is also a time that allows our brains to detoxify. The space between the brain cells increases while we sleep, allowing cerebrospinal fluid (clear fluid that bathes the brain and spinal cord) to circulate more freely, taking away molecules associated with inflammation.[1] Our brains, in fact, are very busy during sleep.

In the 1950s, graduate student Eugene Aserinsky was doing research on sleep.[2] While using an electroencephalogram (EEG) to record brain-wave activity, he was surprised to discover periods of very active sleep, which have become known as rapid eye movement (REM) sleep. Further study with the EEG showed that there are two main types of sleep:

1. Non-REM (NREM), known as quiet sleep

2. REM sleep, known as active sleep, when we can have vivid dreams

We now know that sleep has many stages and cycles, just like a washing machine. And like your clothes, your body needs to go through the whole cycle. If you interrupt the cycle too early, the laundry's not quite clean. Similarly, if you interrupt your sleep cycle too soon, the body doesn't have a chance to completely rest and rejuvenate. There are four stages of sleep. We usually cycle through each of these stages four to five times throughout the night, but we don't necessarily progress through the stages in order.

NREM Stage 1 is a five- to ten-minute period of very light sleep that begins the cycle as we transition from wakefulness to sleep. (Trouble falling asleep can make this stage longer than usual.) The brain waves in this stage are active (but slower than brain waves when we're awake) and they're known as theta waves. During this stage, our heart rate, breathing, and eye movements slow down and our muscles are relaxed with occasional twitches.

NREM Stage 2 is a period of light sleep during which brain-wave activity becomes more rhythmic and we may be less aware of our surroundings. It lasts for about twenty minutes. During this stage, our body temperature decreases, our heart rate slows down more, and our breathing becomes slower and regular. We spend 50–75 percent of our time in this stage, according to the National Sleep Foundation.[3]

NREM Stage 3 is our period of deepest, most restful and restorative sleep. Our brain-wave activity is deep and slow, and we may respond less to noise and activity. During this stage, our muscles relax, our blood pressure drops, and our breathing slows. Some people sleepwalk or wet the bed in this stage. During this physically restful sleep, the body produces growth hormone at the highest levels. It is the most desired sleep phase, helping us wake up refreshed.

REM Sleep is known as "paradoxical sleep" because our brain is at its most active; in fact, our brain-wave activity looks like it does when we're awake. We probably spend about 20 percent of our sleep time in this stage, during which our eyes move rapidly, our breathing speeds up, and our voluntary muscles become immobilized (which may prevent us from acting out our crazy dreams) while our eyes, ears, heart, and diaphragm can still function. Our body temperature stays low during REM sleep as our sex organs become engorged and we dream vividly. As we age, we spend less time in REM sleep.

REM sleep is a very important part of our sleep cycle because, during this stage, cells synthesize proteins that help us to build memory and improve the connections between neural circuits in the brain. REM sleep also helps regulate mood and consolidate memories of events that occurred in the day, though we often see what is not really there. For example, in this stage of sleep we visualize ourselves leaping over tall bridges and fighting with mammoth tigers, but these images don't have a specific location and time and people can morph and disappear without warning. This phase of sleep resembles a psychotic state of hallucinations and delusions, during which our neurons are firing chaotically and not following their usual patterns of emotional correlation.

Only after we wake up does our conscious brain try to stitch together the pieces of our dreams and attach meaning to them. Although dreams can occur in the non-REM sleep cycles, especially NREM stage 2, only in REM sleep do we face the full force of the unimaginable. In other words, the impulses controlled by our prefrontal cortex when we are awake are unleashed during REM sleep. Even though many people don't recall their dreams in this phase, it doesn't mean they didn't dream during REM sleep.

UNDERSTANDING STRESS HORMONES AND DISORDERED SLEEP

Scientific research has confirmed that sleep is as important to our well-being as healthy foods, pure water, and exercise.[4] Yet, when did you last jump out of bed full of energy after a good night's sleep? For most of us, it's been a while. School-aged kids need about 9.5 hours of sleep per night and adults need six to eight hours,[5] but medical research shows that most people are getting less than six hours of sleep a night. The quality of that sleep is as important as the quantity, and many people are getting neither because of disordered sleep.

How Stress Affects Our Sleep

A sleep disorder is different from regular sleeplessness, which affects most people from time to time. Eat or drink too much before bed? Have an important presentation in the morning? Those are common reasons that people experience occasional, situational sleeplessness. But when that sleeplessness becomes habitual, or chronic, it can become a sleep disorder. The stress hormones cortisol and adrenaline activate various arousal centers in the brain and wreak havoc with our normal circadian rhythms and biological clocks. The brain thinks it is being stimulated for a call to action and produces chemicals that cause alertness.

When it comes to the role of the stress hormone cortisol, we couldn't live without it. However, it has its time and place. Under normal circumstances, our cortisol levels gradually build when we're sleeping soundly during the night so we wake bright-eyed and bushy-tailed with peak cortisol levels. This cortisol surge, along with a boost of adrenaline, is a wake-up call for the body. But when we're chronically stressed and hyperaroused, that wake-up call can continue to take place during our regular sleeping hours—causing us to wake up suddenly all alert at 3 a.m. when everyone around us is in REM sleep.

A tense encounter with a co-worker, the death of a loved one, a fight with a partner, or worry about an upcoming event can trigger anxiety and stress that keep us awake. Not all sleep disruptions are related to stress, however. For example, people who travel frequently across time zones disrupt their normal body clock. Shift workers often experience circadian rhythm disorders because their "nights" and "days" are constantly being altered. And artificial light has disrupted our natural circadian rhythms by extending our "days" and shortening our "nights." Artificial light at bedtime, especially blue light from electronic devices, can disrupt melatonin production and make it difficult to wind down. Light hitting the retina at the back of the eye, which usually occurs in the morning, can communicate to the brain that it is time to rev up. It signals wakefulness.

Many people with trouble sleeping seem to think that if they lounge in bed for longer, half-awake and half-asleep, they will increase the amount of sleep they get and be better off. Others think if they do this a few days a week, they can make up for their accumulated sleep debt. While the brain can naturally determine whether to expand or delay the sleep-wake cycle, more time lying in bed not sleeping will not make up for poor-quality sleep. Regardless of the reason, chronic disrupted sleep leads to an abnormal cortisol secretion pattern. When cortisol is disordered, we get an inappropriate surge of this hormone at night when we don't need a heightened level of alertness. Moreover, excessive cortisol at the wrong time and wrong place can disrupt the whole hormone symphony, both day and night, and set us up for obesity, diabetes, and hypertension in the future.

In the short term, we must also consider cortisol and chronic pain as a sleep disruptor. The medical world knows well the famous triad of pain, anxiety, and insomnia, and patients can move through this cycle for years without getting proper treatment. Pain and anxiety travel along the same neural pathway and cause a release of stress hormones that results in insomnia. The lack of sleep delays healing and promotes more pain and anxiety, creating a vicious cycle.

➤ My Story

After my car accident, I experienced many years of chronic pain that prevented me from sleeping or healing properly. Pain creates chemicals for anxiety. Anxiety increases pain sensitivity and causes hyperarousal, which leads to insomnia. Insomnia increases pain sensitivity. This vicious cycle of pain, anxiety, and insomnia quickly becomes a complex set of symptoms. But rather than prescribing sleeping pills, addressing the root cause of the pain is the better solution.

Acupuncture, massage, and occasionally medications helped address my physical pain, but it was visualization and mindfulness techniques to breathe through the pain that made the difference for a better night's sleep. Deep breathing was very helpful to initiate the process. Alternately contracting and relaxing my muscles helped my body to feel heavy and relaxed on the bed at night. Focusing on a word helped to distract my brain and interrupt the stream of constant pain signals. I used the power of mind to create an effect of "remembered wellness." Once I could reimagine myself with a pain-free body, I was able to work toward that goal. It was the breath, mind, word (BMW) meditation and not medication that helped to transform my chronic pain and my sleep! With my mind, brain, and body collaborating, I began to produce more endorphins (natural painkillers), serotonin (antidepressant, antianxiety hormone), and melatonin (natural sleeping pill).

As the quality of my sleep improved, my body began to repair and heal. With less cortisol flowing through my body, my sensitivity to pain decreased, my body and brain were better able to relax, and my quality and quantity of sleep began to normalize.

←·——→

A LACK OF sleep increases stress, and stress and a lack of sleep can create anxiety. Here are a few of the most common sleep disorders that result from this cycle.

➤ Sleep Deprivation and Insomnia

Sleep deprivation is the lack of opportunity to sleep due to external forces such as exams, a new baby, a work schedule, or too much noise or bright light. You don't have the time or right opportunity to induce sleep. In contrast, insomnia is the inability to get enough sleep or enough high-quality sleep despite having plenty of opportunity. The key word to distinguish these conditions is "opportunity" to sleep.[6] We classify insomnia as difficulty falling asleep, difficulty staying asleep, and/or early-morning awakenings. Insomnia can be acute or become chronic, and some people can experience all types of insomnia concurrently.

Insomnia affects about one-third of adults and children,[7] though most cases are undertreated or undiagnosed. This is a very disturbing trend in young children because their developing brain tissue is highly sensitive. Insomnia can be caused by brain stimulants like coffee, alcohol, or drugs or by medical issues such as sleep apnea or restless legs syndrome (see below). It can be caused by too much screen time before bed— researchers have concluded that radiation and light from cell phone screens contributes to insomnia.[8] Age also affects both quality and quantity of sleep. Infants sleep a good part of the day to boost their growth and development, and teenagers sleep a lot, especially when they experience huge growth spurts during puberty, but as we reach age forty, our sleep cycles become shorter and more disrupted. The incidence of insomnia goes up after age fifty and continues to increase with age. We still need the same six to eight hours of sleep but we seem to spend less time in deep and REM sleep.

Psychological reasons, however, account for roughly 50 percent of the cases in which people are diagnosed with insomnia.[9] Sleep surveys reveal we often blame work, technology, kids, pain, diet, medication, alcohol, etc., yet one of the most common factors for insomnia is stress. Contributing factors are depression, anxiety, or a psychophysiological issue in which the idea of sleep or the bedroom itself becomes associated with intense anxiety about getting enough rest. The relationship between stress and insomnia is significant because stress may lead to a lack of sleep, but this lack of sleep also contributes to a number of physical and emotional problems ranging from weight gain to depression.

➤ Obstructive Sleep Apnea

Approximately 90 million Americans snore, and it is the most common cause of sleep disruption.[10] Very loud snoring associated with gasping or stopped breathing (sometimes it can stop for sixty seconds) often indicates obstructive sleep apnea (OSA). This serious condition, which is diagnosed in a sleep lab, can occur when the airway is partially or completely blocked due to obesity or genetic variations of the mouth and airways. When breathing is paused, the level of oxygen saturation in the blood drops to very low levels that trigger the brain to cause a brief awakening, disrupting the normal sleep cycle. If these disruptions are frequent, they cause fatigue, daytime sleepiness, and difficulties in job performance. OSA is also strongly correlated with hypertension, among other chronic diseases. Using a continuous positive airway pressure (CPAP) ventilator can be quite effective to keep the airway open and ensure proper sleep.

➤ Restless Legs Syndrome

If you wake up with an irresistible urge to move your limbs or with tingling, itching, or aching in your legs at night or when you relax, you may be suffering from restless legs syndrome (RLS), also known as Willis-Ekbom disease. About 10 percent of the population in North America and Europe suffers from this neurological disorder, and its prevalence appears to increase with age. Some people attribute RLS to low levels of iron in the brain, whereas others say it may be a result of a dopamine imbalance. There is also a theory that it may have a genetic component.[11] RLS symptoms seem to get worse with anxiety and overwhelm, and alcohol may also trigger RLS in some cases. Treatment includes managing stress through meditation, avoiding alcohol, and using prescription remedies in severe cases.

$$\longleftrightarrow$$

DISRUPTED SLEEP IS also associated with many health concerns:

➤ Fatigue

One of the most common questions I hear from patients is, "Why am I so tired?" Disordered sleep can certainly lead people to feel they are "dead tired all the time" and have "no energy," but not all fatigue results from sleep issues. Fatigue can be a lack of physical or mental energy or capacity for endurance. It is different from drowsiness, which is how we feel after we wake up from a nap or a poor night's sleep. Low energy is often accompanied by apathy and low motivation, and it can result from low thyroid levels, anemia, viral infections, and diseases such as diabetes, heart disease, and chronic obstructive pulmonary disease (COPD). It can also be the result of using cough medications and decongestants, if they interrupt sleep.

Fatigue is very often a symptom of chronic stress, however. For example, lifestyle factors such as a lack of exercise, alcohol use, poor diet, constant travel, and shift work can be the cause of fatigue. And ongoing fatigue can lead to disordered sleep. For example, an overactive hypothalamic-pituitary axis (HPA) can disrupt the normal sleep cycle, increase pain sensitivity, and change neurotransmitters so they cause the brain to be aroused at night and fatigued during the day. To understand whether your fatigue is linked to stress, ask your integrative doctor to look at your cortisol function, circadian rhythms, and adrenal function. Remember, the inner part of the adrenal glands produces norepinephrine and epinephrine, the hormones that regulate the fight-or-flight reaction in the body. Chronic stress can wear down your adrenal function, and the inability to properly put on the brakes can lead to constant fatigue.

➤ Hormonal Fluctuations

Lack of proper sleep affects our sex hormones, and changes in our sex hormones affect our sleep. The cortisol that accompanies stress is the biggest bully on the block. When it surges along hormonal pathways in the body, particularly at night, it prevents other hormones from traveling those pathways and getting where they need to go. The effects, however, are slightly different in men and women.

Men produce most of their testosterone at night and need at least three hours of sleep to reach peak testosterone production during sleeping hours. Thus, inadequate sleep over a prolonged period of time in men is associated with lower levels of testosterone, which has a negative impact on healthy aging and contributes to low energy, reduced libido, poor concentration, and fatigue.[12] Low levels of testosterone also cause a redistribution of body fat, reduce muscle mass and bone density, and depress mood.

In women, fluctuations in hormone levels affect sleep profoundly. Just before her period, a woman's progesterone and estrogen levels drop, which decreases the amount of REM sleep she has. Severe hormone swings due to premenstrual syndrome (PMS) or during perimenopause reduce the level of melatonin production, further contributing to sleep disruptions. In contrast, many pregnant women experience hypersomnia (excessive sleep). They sleep more and experience fatigue. The higher levels of progesterone in the body at that time may contribute to daytime drowsiness, especially in the first trimester.

After many years of looking after menopausal women, I can say that disordered sleep affects most middle-aged women. The changes in body temperature with hot flashes and night sweats contribute to disrupted sleep cycles. Women of reproductive age in high-stress jobs sometimes stop having periods because the excessive cortisol has hijacked the hormonal pathway, and the progesterone needed for proper ovulation just can't get through. Many women state that oral progesterone therapy improves their sleep patterns, reducing fatigue, improving focus, and boosting their mood.

Case Study: Sarah

Sarah, a schoolteacher, came to my clinic complaining that lack of sleep was making her constantly cranky with her husband and her students and that she was so drowsy on her drive home from work, she was worried about falling asleep at the wheel. She told me that she had a longstanding history of insomnia that dated to childhood, but that in the past year, her disrupted sleep had become so severe that she was unable to fall asleep or stay asleep. She was taking antihistamines and drinking two to three glasses of wine in the evenings to help her relax before bed.

Initially, I gave her handouts on sleep hygiene and encouraged her to keep a sleep diary to record her sleep habits. I counseled her about using controlled breathing and meditation to relax her body and advised her to stop using alcohol, which is a stimulant.

After six weeks, she reported that she had used the sleep meditation and breathing techniques daily, stopped drinking alcohol at night, and cut out the antihistamines. She was feeling more relaxed, she said, but her irritability and insomnia before her period were worse than ever. Given her age and the timing of her symptoms, I suspected that Sarah might be perimenopausal and I ordered hormone testing. Sure enough, her progesterone levels were low.

Three months later, she reported that taking oral progesterone pills for two weeks each month had stabilized her mood, eliminated her premenstrual symptoms, and helped her look forward to sleep. We had found the root cause of her insomnia, and the combination of progesterone therapy, controlled meditative breathing, and better sleep hygiene had allowed her to cultivate a healthy sleep mindset for the first time in her life. Knowing that BMW meditation (page 82) had helped her relax, Sarah even shared the technique with her students in the classroom, so they could better regulate their own moods and emotions.

➤ Weight Gain and Obesity

Cortisol cues our body to break down fat cells and move them into the bloodstream to supply energy for the fight-or-flight reaction. If we aren't burning fat cells through exercise, cortisol cues them to be stored in the fat tissue around the belly, so stress plays a huge role in weight gain by changing the hormones that affect our desire to eat or make us feel full.

Ghrelin and leptin are hormones that help regulate our hunger center in the brain. Ghrelin stimulates hunger, while leptin inhibits hunger. Together, they make sure that you manage your energy and get enough food. Ghrelin is produced by the lining in our stomach and is increased by lack of sleep. No wonder sleep-deprived individuals feel hungry all the time and have increased carb cravings. Leptin is secreted abundantly by fat cells at night and is decreased by a lack of sleep. So we tend to overeat when we're sleep deprived because we have less leptin to tell us when we feel full. Excessive cortisol further disrupts leptin and ghrelin. That's three strikes, all due to disrupted sleep and all contributing to weight gain and obesity.

Research indicates that the hormone most implicated in obesity is insulin. Every time we eat, the pancreas produces insulin to help us metabolize our food. Carbohydrates and excess proteins break down into glucose, and insulin helps to store that glucose in the liver for short-term energy use and in the fat cells for longer-term energy use. Normal sleep helps to increase insulin sensitivity, which means the body needs less insulin to do its job efficiently. A chronic lack of sleep, however, increases insulin resistance, which can lead to obesity and type 2 diabetes. Obesity researchers now generally agree that insulin resistance is the main culprit for weight gain, especially fat deposits around the belly, and is related to abnormal levels of cortisol. Proper sleep is therefore important when addressing weight loss, diabetes, fatigue, and overall health.

➤ Low Mood, Poor Concentration,
  and Lack of Adaptability

We have all experienced waking up after a poor night's sleep feeling cranky, overtired, foggy, and even aggressive. Besides changing our hormones, cortisol causes changes in our neurotransmitters, the brain chemicals that determine mood, mental clarity, focus, and sleep. When cortisol peaks in the morning, we are more alert for the coming day, our mind is clear, and we feel more motivated. Researchers in Germany found that subjects who had adequate sleep were much better at learning adaptive behavior.[13] Based on this information, researchers established that sleep helps the brain stay balanced and improves its "synaptic plasticity." That is, neurons are better able to adapt to new conditions when we have enough sleep.

The researchers also found that certain areas of the brain are more sensitive to sleep deprivation than others are. Problem-solving and concentration centers are slower to react in sleep-deprived patients. Poor retention and slower recall affect our cognitive ability. In other words, lack of sleep impairs attention, alertness, reaction time, memory, and reasoning skills. On the other hand, a good sleep strengthens creative thinking. Many scientists and inventors have had their best ideas while sleeping. Make sure you get your shut-eye; you may wake up smarter than when you went to sleep!

➤ Immune System Function and Sleep

Sleep deprivation takes a toll on your immune system. In the early stages of sleep, T cells, which float around in the blood looking for damaged tissue or foreign invaders, peak in concentration and enhance the body's ability to form an initial immune response. As we'll see in the next chapter, skimping on sleep causes an imbalance in the immune system, leaving the whole body at risk for infection and disease.

HOW TO CULTIVATE A HEALTHY SLEEP MINDSET

From special pillows to unique sheets, white-noise machines to aromatherapy oils, over-the-counter medicines to herbs and potions, the marketplace is exploding with aids to help people get a good night's sleep. You can even hire a sleep coach! Americans spent about $41 billion on sleep aids and remedies, not including over-the-counter medications, in 2015 and that figure is expected to rise to $52 billion by 2020.[14] The truth is that our mind is one of our most powerful allies in getting a good night's sleep and it's not going to cost you any money.

It is normal and acceptable to experience sleeplessness from time to time. In our clinic, for example, we see many patients who have adapted their sleep-wake cycles to fit their work schedules. And most of us have experienced a night or two of poor sleep after a long flight across several time zones. However, our bodies are designed to adapt only occasionally, not constantly.

Sleep specialists have found that most patients suffering from sleep disorders have negative belief systems about sleep, and many of those patients also have varying degrees of anxiety. Research has revealed that most people have a unique sleep threshold at which they can fall into a normal sleep. Those who have a low threshold for sleep, possibly set at birth or in childhood, are easily thrown off balance by even minor stress. Insomnia follows quickly until they resolve the stressor and re-establish their normal threshold. The good news is that if negative mindsets such as, "Sleep is a waste of time," or "I can function on four hours of sleep" can create our poor sleep behavior, then we can learn techniques that calm the body, slow brain-wave activity at bedtime, and create a more positive sleep mindset. This approach, combined with excellent sleep hygiene, is the basis for a good night's sleep.

Reclaim Your Rest

A good way to re-set your nervous system to rest-and-digest mode before bedtime is to incorporate a relaxation ritual before going to sleep. Some people find that having a hot bath, reading for a few minutes, or listening to soothing music are helpful for slowing down the racing mind and relaxing the muscles. Stress and sleep are closely linked, and using relaxation techniques addresses both issues. I like to combine breathing and mindful meditation (see the Breath, Mind, Word Method, page 82) with visualization and sleep hypnosis.

Sleep hypnosis is a powerful exercise I use with patients to change their subconscious mindset. Sleep, like hypnosis, is an altered state of consciousness. Use the first stage of sleep to embed constructive visualizations aimed at helping you sleep. Imagine yourself falling into a deep, restful slumber using all your senses. Our mind loves imagery, so begin with watching yourself relaxing your muscles and feeling comfortable. Your body weighs down the mattress as you drift off to a deep sleep. Then imagine yourself sleeping through the night. Use your senses to create a picture of you waking up full of energy and vitality after a fabulous night of sleep.

Guided imagery or visualization techniques help to connect our conscious mind with the subconscious so we can regain control over automatic negative thoughts and guide the body to more desirable behavior. The beauty of this technique is that it can be customized for different patients with different goals. For example, Dr. Leora Kuttner, a pediatric psychologist, uses it to help distract teens undergoing painful bone marrow implants so that they require fewer chemicals to manage pain. She has patients imagine that the needle is injecting a beautiful golden healing liquid that is eating up all the cancer cells like a video game. Similarly, many professional athletes use this technique to imagine themselves winning a competition, to the point they can feel the medal around their neck and hear the roaring crowds. When we use it for sleep, we imagine being in a state of deep, restful sleep.

To begin, lie down in a calm, quiet place. Imagine yourself floating on a serene lake, peacefully staring at the beautiful blue sky while being rocked gently by warm waves. Enlist all your senses to fully imagine the sights, sounds, smells, and sensations of the experience. Or picture yourself walking quietly along a sandy beach, feeling the fine, soft sand beneath your feet as the warm ocean breeze blows through your hair and the setting sun casts a warm glow on your face. Whatever your calming image, allow yourself to be transported there.

If you are having trouble getting started, try the app mySleepButton, which has you form a mental image of benign objects (for example, picture a pen or picture a car) every few seconds. For meditation, I often recommend Headspace, or the apps Buddhify and Insight Timer. New research also suggests that soundwave technology can encourage sleep.[15] Binaural beats are audio files in which the listener hears a different frequency in each ear. The brain actually perceives a single tone that is the difference between the two frequencies and "tunes" to it, a process called entrainment. By manipulating the frequency patterns, scientists can affect the level of arousal in the brain. Binaural beats for sleep therapy use four frequency patterns, each designed to simulate one of the four phases of sleep.

If you decide to try using video and/or audio apps, dim your screen and use headphones to minimize the distractions of light and sound. And work toward visualizing sleep and guiding meditation on your own. Do this for twenty-one nights to establish sleep neural pathways so your body becomes conditioned. Act as if deep, restful sleep has already happened.

TRY THESE ADDITIONAL STEPS, alone or in combination, to reclaim your rest.

➤ Improve Your Sleep Hygiene
Light, sound, and other stimulants can impair sleep, so try to limit these factors to improve the quality of your sleep. Eye

shades and earplugs can help block light and sound if you're trying to sleep on an airplane or in a noisy room. When you go to bed, try putting your phone in another room rather than on your night table. Let your friends, family, and work colleagues know you are not a 9-1-1 responder on call all the time and avoid the temptation to answer texts or phone calls. Repeat the phrase, "I am not responsible for everyone" like a mantra.

The key to improving your sleep hygiene is to tailor it to your individual needs. If you have rituals and habits that help to calm you down and create a good environment for sleep, make time for them. Rearrange your bedroom if you need to; find another space for your computer, your pet, or your baby; introduce candles or incense or soft music; replace your pillow and buy cool, comfortable bed linens—do whatever it takes to be relaxed and comfortable when you go to sleep. If you're in the habit of smoking or drinking too much caffeine or alcohol late in the day, make a conscious effort to change those routines to improve your sleep. Also try to avoid stimulants in medications, such as pseudoephedrine in cold remedies, that cause the brain to be more hyperaroused and disrupt the sleep-wake cycle. Instead, make time for regular exercise and create rituals such as stretching before bedtime to cue the body that it's time to rest.

➤ Use Cognitive Behavioral Therapy for Insomnia

Dr. Rob Comey is a psychiatrist who specializes in sleep disorders and treats many of my patients. He recommends cognitive behavioral therapy (CBT) to address specific disorders, such as anxiety, depression, phobias, and addictions. Cognitive behavioral therapy for insomnia (CBT-I) teaches you to recognize and change the beliefs that cause insomnia, and it can be helpful when anxiety or fear is keeping you awake. The idea is to reframe or eliminate the negative thoughts and worries that keep you from falling asleep.

Sometimes your sleep specialist may have you take a biofeedback device home to record your daily activity to help identify patterns that affect sleep. The behavioral part of CBT-I helps you develop good sleep habits and avoid behaviors that keep you from sleeping well, and these can be customized to your particular situation. Depending on the severity of your sleep problems, your therapist may recommend some of the following CBT-I techniques.

Controlled Stimulus Therapy (CST) is a form of classical conditioning in which the goal is to strengthen (or re-establish) the link between the bed and sleep and to weaken the learned association between the bed and wakefulness, worry, fear, frustration, and anxiety. To do this, you remove the negative external factors in your bedroom that are easy to change: minimize light exposure, keep the temperature comfortable, avoid noise, take the TV out of the room. Then, you avoid daytime naps, go to bed only when you are sleepy, and set a consistent wake time. Most importantly, you use your bed for sleep and sex only, rather than lying in bed with your iPad or other digital device. And if you cannot sleep, you get out of bed and do something quiet like reading a book or stretching. Initially, you may spend more time out of bed than in it. But the time you spend in bed will be time spent sleeping. And as you strengthen the link between the bed and sleep, you will begin to spend more time in bed asleep.

Sleep Restriction Therapy (SRT), also known as compressed sleep or sleep consolidation, is another form of classical conditioning. Again, the goal is to strengthen (or re-establish) the link between the bed and sleep and to weaken the learned association between the bed and wakefulness, worry, fear, frustration, and anxiety. With this technique, you determine the total number of hours you are actually sleeping each night and allow yourself only that amount of time in bed. Instead of lying in bed tossing and turning while your brain creates dialogues of negativity, you stay out of the bedroom and awake until your "new" bedtime: the one that gives you just your actual number of sleeping hours. Both CST and SRT are designed to align your bedtime and rise time with your internal clock.

At first you may struggle to stay awake at night, causing partial sleep deprivation, which makes you more tired during the day. In severe cases where sleep deprivation involves sleepwalking or other unusual behaviors, a sleep specialist may monitor you for safety reasons. Sleep specialist Dr. Rob Comey emphasizes consistency. He suggests you turn out the lights for sleep no earlier than the same specific time every night and get out of bed no later than the same specific time every morning. Once your sleep has improved, your time in bed gradually increases. This technique increases sleep efficiency and causes an increased sleep drive.

Paradoxical Intention Therapy promotes a healthy sleep mindset to induce sleep. Remaining passively awake, also called paradoxical intention, involves avoiding any effort to fall asleep. Because worrying you can't sleep can keep you awake, the idea of this therapy is to take the pressure off. Catastrophic thoughts such as, "I will lose my job," or "Insomnia will kill me" can become ingrained beliefs. Letting go of this worry can help you relax and make it easier to fall asleep. To do this, it helps to upgrade your inner dialogue (page 28) and then tap into your conscious brain (page 55). For example, practice positive self-talk: rather than making a list of things to do tomorrow (which turns on the gas), practice saying, "It will all be there tomorrow and I trust it will get done." This simple phrase shifts the brain from making an urgent to a non-urgent list. Or challenge the belief you can function on less than four hours of sleep. Focus on a more beneficial belief: "My body loves to heal and repair while I sleep," or "I am ensuring vitality and longevity by resting my body for at least seven hours."

➤ Use Sleep Medications Sparingly, If at All

Almost one in three Americans reports problems with sleep, so it isn't surprising that between 2006 and 2011, the number of sleeping pills prescribed in the United States increased from 47 million to 80 million per year.[16] Most of these prescription sleep medications belong to a class of drugs called benzodiaze-pines or similar chemicals that target the gamma-aminobutyric acid (GABA) receptors in the brain. These receptors sedate or tranquilize the central nervous system. Benzodiazepines are not that effective for curing insomnia because the brain becomes tolerant of their effect after just a few weeks of use. Studies show that they increase sleep time by, on average, only twelve minutes a night, and they may not increase sleep quality either. Most sleeping pills, such as the most commonly prescribed zopiclone, are for short-term use only. All of these drugs are dependence-forming, may lead to addiction, and may cause memory loss with prolonged use.

Common side effects of sleeping pills include daytime seda-tion and confusion, and if mixed with alcohol, these effects last longer than usual. The side effects are often more pronounced in older people, because they're more likely to have a low body weight and slower metabolism, and the sleeping pills may negatively interact with other medications. Seniors report memory problems and even difficulty with balance after taking benzodiazepines, and the incidence of hip fractures is higher among those who complain of dizziness and loss of balance. In fact, some people who take sleep medications experience worse insomnia after they stop, an effect known as rebound insomnia.

Addressing the lack of sleep is important, and resorting to the occasional sleep aid is better than chronic sleep deprivation. However, even with all the strides we have made in medicine, we haven't come up with the ideal sleeping pill that effectively restores a normal sleep cycle yet has minimal side effects. I don't recommend treating young children with sleeping pills at all. Instead, setting good sleep routines and providing tools for sensible sleep behaviors at an early age can set the stage for healthy sleep cycles as adults. Establishing this baseline threshold for sleep, as it is known, can be one of the best gifts we give our children. For adults, I only recommend sleep medications as the solution of last resort once your physician has investigated the causes for your lack of sleep and exhausted all other treatments. And if you find yourself dependent on sleeping pills for sleep, then it is best to taper off these medications slowly while determining the root cause of your sleep difficulties and developing healthier sleep routines.

The Benefits of a Healthy Sleep Mindset

If there's an upside to the increase in insomnia and sleep disorders, it's that researchers have been encouraged to better understand our sleep-wake cycle and look for better solutions to disrupted sleep. Consequently, we have many more options for using the mind to cultivate healthier attitudes toward sleep. When we sleep better, our overall health is improved in very important ways. Sleep makes you more alert, improves your memory, and optimizes cognitive function. And perhaps most importantly, sleep reduces our stress levels, which reduces inflammation; decreases our chances of major illnesses such as obesity, heart disease, and cancer; and improves our mood. Best of all, adequate sleep allows the body to naturally heal and repair itself, so we can keep living our healthiest lives.

CONCLUSION

In my years of practice, insomnia has been one of the most challenging complaints to address. Most prescription drugs come with a huge list of side effects. While the burgeoning sleep-aid industry promotes the use of over-the-counter remedies, natural herbs, and relaxation apps, my clinical experience shows that good sleep comes down to cultivating a "sleep mindset" and consistent sleep habits. Some natural supplements (Appendix B) can be helpful when we are trying to establish good sleep routines, and audio apps can be a good tool to monitor our sleep and help improve sleep cycles by cueing the brain to slow down and prepare for sleep. We do not have substantial data on the effectiveness of these, but there are many anecdotal cases where people have found some supplements and apps helpful.

Sleep is vital to our well-being! From our electrical brain waves to the chemicals and hormones of our cellular biology, sleep is essential to every system in the body. If you think you can burn the candle at both ends by getting up early and staying up late to get ahead, think again. We would all perform better, be happier and more energetic, and even look and feel a little sexier if we had enough quality sleep.

8.

Mind Your Immune System

Natural forces within us are the true healers of disease.
Hippocrates

SELF-ASSESSMENT

Our immune system keeps us healthy so we can enjoy life and avoid living with constant infections and inflammation. When we aren't healthy, our poor quality of life challenges us and keeps us from doing the things we enjoy and find fulfilling. Relaxing and having fun feels nearly impossible. The severe symptoms of immune dysfunction can be debilitating. When it comes to stress, the immune system is particularly sensitive yet we don't usually make that connection.

Do you:

· get frequent infections, such as pneumonia, bronchitis, or sinus, ear, or skin infections?

- often deal with inflammation and joint problems?

- have blood disorders, such as low platelet counts or anemia?

- suffer digestive problems, such as cramping, loss of appetite, nausea, and diarrhea?

- suffer from cold hands or dry eyes?

- often feel fatigued?

- deal with stiff joints or muscle aches?

- deal with food sensitivities and allergies?

- experience symptoms of hay fever: runny nose, itchy eyes, and sneezing?

- have problems with skin conditions such as eczema or psoriasis?

Our immune system has been a work in progress for millions of years. While initially efficient, over the millennia it has become a multilayered, complex, and precision-driven system. The immune response defends us from our environment, thus it is on constant surveillance 24/7, scanning the body for threatening invaders. It begins to protect us when we are newly born and continues to add to its memory bank as we get older, so it can respond to all past exposures as well as new ones. It's a 9-1-1 emergency system, the first responder to rescue and repair tissues and cells in danger.

For years, we attributed problems with the immune system to external factors such as toxins or infections. We now know that genetics, environment, maternal immunity, diet, and stress management all play a role in creating a healthy immune system and that some of these factors are under our control. When the immune system becomes hyperresponsive and begins to harm the body it is supposed to protect, we can optimize our diet and our gut function, and especially manage our stress to minimize the damage.

Our state of mind has both direct and indirect impacts on the function of our immune system. Negative beliefs and thoughts turn on the sympathetic nervous system (SNS)—the gas—and directly compromise the immune system.[1] We know that when produced in excessive amounts for a long time, stress hormones cause a significant disruption to gut function. And since 80 percent of the immune system is in the gut, both local and systemic inflammation caused by stress or poor diet predispose the body to immune problems. In contrast, when we engage our parasympathetic nervous system (PNS)—the brakes—it promotes a stronger immune response. It is no surprise, then, that happier, less-stressed people often have a healthier, more robust immune system.

THE IMMUNE SYSTEM 101

The immune system is a layered network of defense mechanisms to protect the body against tiny infection-causing organisms such as bacteria, viruses, parasites, and fungi. Given that the body is warm and has a ready supply of nutrients in the bloodstream, it provides the ideal environment for microorganisms to grow and replicate. Foreign infectious agents thrive under these conditions and therefore try to break down the body's barriers to take advantage of this environment and multiply. The immune system, therefore, evolves as our external environment changes and produces new forms of organisms that find new ways to breach our existing defense systems. I like to think of the body's immune system as an army defending against foreign invaders.

The key to a healthy immune system is its remarkable ability to distinguish between the body's own cells (self) and foreign cells (nonself). The body's immune defenses coexist peacefully with cells that carry distinctive "self" marker molecules. We often refer to this ability as immune tolerance. Specific immune defense cells will ignore the body's own tissues as well as proteins circulating in the blood that they have seen before. When immune defenders encounter cells or organisms carrying unrecognizable markers, they go into attack mode, because this sensitive system recognizes a foreign substance as a "foe."

The immune system is a complex topic that doctors and medical students often struggle with! Psychoneuroimmunology is the study of interactions among the brain and the endocrine and immune systems of the body. The brain communicates with the immune system through the autonomic nervous system (ANS) and neuroendocrine activity. Both pathways generate signals that the immune system perceives by way of receptors on the surface of lymphocytes and other immune cells. An activated immune system generates chemical signals (cytokines) that are perceived by the nervous system. Next I describe the key components of this bidirectional communication system.

The Origins of Immunity

An infant is born with a small army of immune factors to prepare for the germ-filled world. Starting in the early stages of pregnancy, the bone marrow of the fetus manufactures lines of white cells that will learn to attack infectious agents. Throughout pregnancy, but especially in the last three months, mothers are passing along immune antibodies to the baby through the placenta. Antibodies are like tiny heat-seeking missiles that circulate in the blood, targeting foreign and dangerous substances. The mother is able to pass on her defenses to the baby during pregnancy. This is called *passive immunity*, because the baby didn't manufacture these antibodies.

Regardless of whether a baby is born vaginally or by caesarean section, it receives immune support from the mother after birth if she breastfeeds. Breast milk provides passive immunity first through colostrum, known as first milk, which contains large numbers of immune cells. The white blood cells in colostrum are essential in helping to eliminate harmful bacteria for the infant before its own production line is ready. Breast milk contains a lot of antibodies called immunoglobulins, which help line the baby's gut to protect it from germs. Besides antibodies, breast milk contains various molecules such as chains of sugars called oligosaccharides that help to neutralize bacteria. Free fatty acids and certain proteins also assist the immune system by limiting the growth of bacteria and viruses in the baby's gut. The composition of this first human microbiome exposure has long-lasting effects on the development and effectiveness of the immune system. Again, we call this form of immunity passive, since the baby's immune system is not making but simply receiving the antibodies. Blood transfusions are another form of passive immunity.

During and after birth, infants also develop their own immunity from external sources. We call this ability to manufacture antibodies and fight infections *active immunity*. In babies born through vaginal childbirth, it begins with exposure to the mother's resident vaginal and intestinal bacteria, which helps to inoculate the sterile gut of the baby. This "immune education," or imprinting, is essential for future health and reduces the likelihood of developing autoimmune diseases, since immune cells need training on how to protect the body from harm before we no longer have the maternal antibodies. With a caesarean section delivery, this direct contact is absent, so bacteria in the environment become the source for the infant's gut colonization.

Both the mental and physical health of a pregnant mother contributes to the well-being of the developing baby. Research published in *Brain, Behavior, and Immunity*[2] shows that infants born to mothers with pre- and postnatal depression had lower levels of an important immune antibody in the first few months of life. The immune system undergoes a lot of adaptation during pregnancy, and stress hormones in the mother may result in babies with lower levels of antibodies, which makes them more likely to have allergies. Chronic prenatal stress causes other dysfunctions in the baby's immune system too, including changes to cells in the bone marrow and developing white cells, and alterations to inflammation markers. The mother's levels of cortisol and adrenaline pose a threat to developing organs of the infant's immune system.

Stress hormones affect breast milk production, as well. A mother in stressful circumstances releases more cortisol and adrenaline, which may reduce the amount of milk she produces and make her more agitated and less likely to nurse her baby. Cortisol crosses the blood barrier and enters breast milk, and studies show that "secondary cortisol" may cause more agitation and crying in babies. Cortisol may also enter a baby's gastrointestinal tract, changing the neurotransmitters that enter the brain. Stressed babies may stress their immune system, though research is pending on the exact effects of secondary cortisol.

After the first few months of life, we acquire most of our immunity by actively manufacturing our own antibodies to fight foreign bacteria and viruses. When the body encounters a foreign antigen—a microorganism such as a virus or a food such as a peanut, really anything that can trigger an immune response—it recognizes the antigen and develops specific antibodies for it. Then, when the body encounters the virus or bacteria in the outside world, the body has learned to fight off that antigen and we don't succumb to the virus. This immunity can last a lifetime.

We know that exposure to diverse germs plays a large role in training the immune system to develop resistance to disease in later life. In fact, children exposed to other children, pets, and dirt have a more robust immune system and less chance of developing hay fever than those who are not. In the contemporary Western world, our focus on cleanliness—and abundant use of disinfectants and antiseptic wipes—may be doing a disservice to children's gut microbiome and consequently to their immune system.

A theory known as the "hygiene hypothesis" was first introduced in the late 1980s in the *British Medical Journal*.[3] The hypothesis states that when children encounter microorganisms, their immune system develops. When exposed to a diverse variety of bacteria at an early age, a child's immune system becomes more robust. Children who are overly protected (living in near-sterile environments) don't get the early exposure and imprinting needed to prime the immune system. Clearly, parents need to ensure that children are not exposed to fecal bacteria or infected meat and that surfaces contaminated by serious infectious agents are cleaned with disinfectant. But just like a bodybuilder trains by gradually exposing their muscles to heavier and heavier weights to build strength, the immune system must train by fighting off everyday germs to be robust and ready to fight the big infection.

Vaccinations use this same strategy. Vaccinations are injections of weakened or inactive pathogens that cause the body to create specific antibodies. For example, we inoculate children against measles and mumps so they are protected when and if they encounter the virus in daily life. Similarly, when we plan to travel abroad, we may get a hepatitis A vaccination to protect us specifically from that virus.

The Immune System as a Three-Tiered Defense System
The immune system comprises distinct organs, tissues, and immune cells that work together like a well-run army (Figure 8.1). Unlike your heart or your brain, the immune system has bases in strategic locations all around the body. The bone marrow, for example, acts as an incubator raising newly formed white blood cells that will join your body's army. The thymus (an immune gland located near our heart) is the barracks, where immune cells are trained and specialized into various types of agents. The skin and mucous membranes are external surveillance sites (like the CIA) where attackers are recognized and the rest of the system is alerted. Finally, the spleen and lymphatic system are internal surveillance sites (like the FBI) where attackers that have already breached the body can be identified and killed.

Once immune cells receive an alarm signal that says "foreign invader," they undergo tactical changes and produce powerful chemicals to launch a counterattack quickly. These chemicals allow the cells to regulate their own growth and behavior, enlist fellow cells, and direct new recruits to areas of trouble. Armed with secretions and cells to wipe out offending agents, the immune system can also recognize and remember millions of different enemies. We can develop immunity to certain antigens or destroy them.

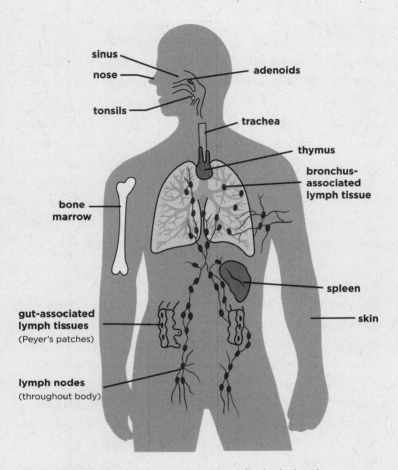

Figure 8.1. The body's immune system (also includes the mucous membranes lining the inner nose, trachea, and gastrointestinal tract)

Communication within the immune system is complex, and this elaborate messaging network is the secret to its success. The amount of information exchanged within the millions and millions of cells is astounding. Like other body systems, our immune system seeks homeostasis (balance). And it has the ability to call upon various levels of defense. It can rely on existing barriers to keep out routine antigens. It can call on an inflammatory response to neutralize an invader that has penetrated the barrier. Or it can mount a quick and lethal full-body response to bring down a more urgent antigen. The whole army can mobilize efficiently to fight with full force and fury.

We've covered the difference between passive and active immunity. Our bodies also possess an *innate* immunity, which is always present. Innate immunity comprises our "first" and "second" lines of defense; they are innate because barriers and the inflammatory response will react to all types of attacks.

➤ First Line of Defense (Barriers)

The immune system prioritizes keeping foreign invaders out by providing surface barriers that don't allow invaders to get inside the body. This form of innate immunity prevents infection from occurring in the first place. Think of this line of defense like a brick-and-mortar wall that keeps germs out physically and chemically. The skin and mucous membranes are the walls of our immune fortress. Our skin is the single largest organ of the body, and it acts as a barrier against many bacteria, viruses, and even toxic chemicals in our environment. It is covered with a protective layer of fats and oils, which act as a repellent. Tiny hairs, layers of protective proteins, and cells line the mucous membranes of our mouth, nose, sinuses, and respiratory tract to keep invaders out. The gut-associated lymphatic tissue (GALT) is the barrier for the immune system in our gastrointestinal tract.

If a rash, infection, or injury breaks our skin barrier, we are at higher risk for infection. For example, the AIDS virus cannot get through normal, intact skin but it can cross over the cells of broken skin, where it replicates and invades the body.

➤ Second Line of Defense (General Infantry)

At the first sign of a breach, the body sends out the general infantry. These nonspecialized cells and antibodies from the innate immune system are the first responders that activate after any threat. They reconnoiter the situation, clear away small numbers of invaders, and shore up the defenses to prevent further unexpected contact. The key here is that these troops respond the same way to every type of infection: they are part of our innate immunity. They don't differentiate between different types of invaders; they just try to quickly eradicate the threat and restore order.

To reiterate, once the invaders are inside the body, our immune system sends out white blood cells to the infection site. It might also release chemicals called cytokines, which are nonspecific proteins that increase blood flow to the area, cause localized swelling, and eliminate the foreign foes. As a final general response, the body might mount a fever, increasing our body temperature to activate proteins to suppress or kill off the unwanted bacteria. All of these changes (redness, swelling, and fever) are known as the inflammatory response.

Local inflammation helps the body protect itself in the area of attack but systemic, or widespread, inflammation is harmful or even deadly. If a rash, infection, or disease overwhelms the general infantry, we become more susceptible to illness, organ damage, or possibly even death.

➤ Third Line of Defense (Tactical Unit)

The final line of defense is specific and includes the cells that produce antibodies to specific antigens. Think of specially trained defense units adapted to particular invaders—paratroopers to get into difficult-to-reach areas of the body, tactical units that can mobilize coordinated attacks in several parts of the body simultaneously—to aggressively attack and destroy foreign invaders and return the body to safety and homeostasis. The immune cells and lymphatic system are the key coordinators of our specific immune response system.

Immune cells can live in the lymph organs, which serve as a home base while waiting for the signal to begin an attack. Lymph organs, spread throughout the body, include the lymph nodes, thymus, spleen, appendix, and tonsils and adenoids. We can sometimes feel small bean-shaped lymph nodes in our neck and armpits or groin. An active lymph node is tender after an infection. It contains cells that have actively fought invaders face to face, and it's on alert to spring into action again if the call comes. Lymphatic fluid is a clear liquid that fills the lymph vessels that connect all the lymph nodes; it bathes the cells and tissues and helps to clear out germs. All immune cells are produced in our bone marrow, which is the training ground for immature white cells destined to become fighter cells called lymphocytes. B cells and T cells are the main types of tactical unit cells.

B cells target antigens circulating in the bloodstream and can make antibodies to fight them. For cough and cold viruses that continue to change and adapt, the B cells need to continually change their strategy to keep up. Thus, our immune system adapts constantly to upgrade its arsenal. Think of B cells as highly trained snipers that are conditioned for only certain terrain. The sniper that specializes in jungle combat won't be able to recognize an attacker hiding in the desert. There are many types of B cells capable of detecting very distinct antigens and creating a specific antibody to each of them. However, B cells cannot penetrate a cell infected by a virus or damaged by cancer.

Think of T cells as the special forces. They don't recognize free-floating antigens, which means they only attack the cells already infected by a virus or distorted by cancer. There are three types of T cells: helper T cells, cytotoxic (killer) T cells, and regulatory T cells. Helper T cells coordinate immune response by communicating with other cells. They can stimulate B cells to produce more antibodies or they can activate another line of killer T cells. Killer T cells directly attack and destroy cells infected by viruses and abnormal cells that may become cancerous. Regulatory T cells call off the immune system attack once the killer T cells conquer the invader. These important mediators have a suppressive effect, ensuring the killer T cells stop killing.

Both B cells and T cells can convert to memory cells after being activated, which is to say that they become dormant but stay in reserve to provide long-term immunity at the appropriate time for a specific antigen.

Immunity is our body's ability to recognize germs and prevent them from causing illness. Our immune system is sensitive and precise, and it knows how to distinguish "self" from "nonself," which is why we often reject organs and tissues from other human donors without the use of drugs to prevent "host rejection." Similarly, we reject foreign proteins from food unless the digestive system breaks them down into parts recognizable by our immune system as food. Inherited genes can influence our immunity, so faced with the same antigen, some people respond forcefully, others feebly, and some not at all. Immunity can be strong or weak, short-lived or long-lasting, depending on the antigen, the amount of antigen, and the route by which it enters the body. However, unmanaged stress can also compromise our immunity and seems to be a common denominator for the prevalence of autoimmune disease.

UNDERSTANDING STRESS HORMONES
AND COMPROMISED IMMUNITY

For years, we attributed disruptions to our immune system—colds and flus, skin rashes, food allergies, arthritis, and so on—to invading organisms (external agents) or to genetic predisposition. We focused on the physical causes of a disease without realizing that our inner beliefs communicate with this intelligent defense system. More recent research teams have referred to the immune system as our "floating brain" because immune cells actively take part in sending chemical messages throughout the body. Our thoughts, moods, sensations, and expectations can be transmitted to our immune cells. In both children and adults, immune problems emerge after chronic stress reaction, and they worsen in stressful situations (Figure 8.2).

How the immune system is altered through the regulation of stress pathways is under further study and new data will emerge. However, we do know that the ANS regulates our immune system, and if immunity is weakened by chronic stress, it cannot fight infection—which leaves the body vulnerable to invading pathogens like viruses or bacteria. Chronic exposure to these antigens allows the immune system no time to rest or "arm" itself again. The immune system therefore remains in a very heightened sense of alert and it will attack everything it sees—even itself.

Our stress hormones cortisol and adrenaline are inflammatory to the immune system through various mechanisms, especially through the gut, as discussed in Chapter 4. As the gut houses 80 percent of the body's immune system, a chronic supply of stress hormones to the gut causes local and systemic inflammation that compromises the body's ability to fight infection. Poor diet, medication, alcohol, and toxin exposure also stress the gut, with the result that our immune system rarely gets downtime. It then goes into hyperresponsive or attack mode with serious repercussions for our health.

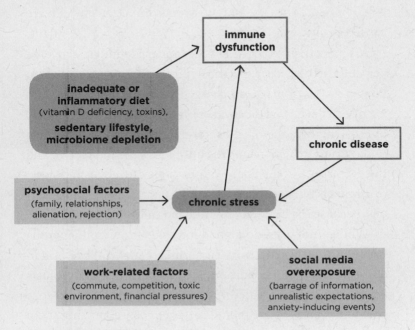

Figure 8.2. How chronic stress contributes to immune dysfunction and chronic disease

How Stress Affects Our Immunity

➤ Antibiotic-Resistant Diseases and Dysbiosis

Antibiotics fight bacterial infections that cause illness or death, such as strep throat, pneumonia, and wound infections. The drugs work by slowing the growth of bacteria or suspending their growth. Since bacteria have a cell wall and human cells do not, these drugs destroy the bacterial cell wall without affecting human cells. When the cell wall is destroyed, the bacteria cannot multiply and the infection is contained. (Antibiotics do not work on viruses, because these infectious agents don't have cell walls. Antibiotics are therefore ineffective for treating the common cold, flus, sore throats, and most sinus infections, which are caused by viruses.)

After Scottish biologist Dr. Alexander Fleming discovered penicillin in 1928, it became widely prescribed and prevented millions of deaths from bacterial infections. Since then, antibiotics have been developed for a wide range of bacteria. Today, many of those highly adaptable bacteria have formed a resistance to the drugs, which means the antibiotics are ineffective and the bacteria continue to grow. Infections caused by antibiotic-resistant bacteria are more difficult to treat and often more serious, because the bacteria grow and multiply unchecked.

While antibiotics do a good job of destroying dangerous bacteria, they also destroy the normal, beneficial bacteria in our gut, creating a condition of imbalance called dysbiosis (page 102). Infants treated with antibiotics show altered composition of bacteria for months after exposure, making them more likely to develop gut problems. We also need to concern ourselves with more than just the antibiotics used to treat bacterial infections. Farm animals and agricultural crops treated with antibiotics can alter our microbiome as well. Data is emerging that the altered microbiome may be linked to inflammation in the brain and to depression.[4] Insulin resistance and weight gain can also result from an altered microbiome.

➤ Autoimmune Diseases
Inflammation is a natural response by the body to help repair damage, kill bacteria, or heal wounds. It is part of our second

line of defense and is designed to provide a quick and dirty way to combat foreign invaders. Signs of inflammation such as swelling and mucous secretions enlist the immune system to deliver a heavy dose of immune cells to the affected area. We couldn't have survived without this defense mechanism because this "superboost" to the body gives us a better chance of survival. However, chronic stress pushes the body into the hypervigilant high-alert phase, which triggers a "hyperinflammatory" chemical response. The lack of rest and recovery means the gut lining doesn't have time to repair and heal. The immune system, therefore, becomes suppressed due to the inflammatory load and the compromised microbiome, and it stages a mutiny.

Autoimmune (AI) disease is an umbrella term for different manifestations of an immune system that has gone rogue and begun to attack itself. It is as if our "army" undergoes a mutiny or a coup, and a rogue faction begins an assault on the home base. For example, instead of targeting pathogens, our B cells can produce antibodies that latch on to "self" cells in our body. In hypothyroidism, the immune system produces antithyroid antibodies that destroy the gland. The body stops producing thyroid hormone, which leads to weight gain, cold intolerance, constipation, dry skin, and more.

Depending on our individual genetics, weakest link, and gut health, AI diseases may show up in the joints, gut, skin, or thyroid. Though you may not have known it, many common and debilitating diseases have autoimmune origins. Among the AI diseases we hear about most often are rheumatoid arthritis, ulcerative colitis, Crohn's disease, psoriasis, lupus, multiple sclerosis, and hypo/hyperthyroidism.

Disease	Autoimmune Target
Rheumatoid arthritis	Joints
Crohn's disease	Gut
Ulcerative colitis	Large intestine
Multiple sclerosis	Nervous system
Type 1 diabetes	Pancreas
Psoriasis	Skin
Hashimoto's disease (Hypothyroid)	Thyroid
Graves' disease (Hyperthyroid)	Thyroid
Lupus	Multiple systems (e.g., joints, skin, kidney)
Myasthenia gravis	Muscles
Vasculitis	Blood vessels

AI diseases affect 35 million people in North America and the numbers continue to grow. New cases are being reported as data is collected, and AI diseases are now the third most commonly diagnosed chronic diseases after cancer and heart disease.[5] Women suffer more often than men—in fact, 78 percent more.[6] In my own practice, I see many young women being diagnosed with lupus and multiple sclerosis—most of them after severe stressors such as a failed marriage, toxic work conditions, or failed university courses. We used to attribute the cause of auto-immune diseases to viruses, genetics, and external agents but we now know that the causes are multifactorial and that stress is a large contributor.

To effectively treat AI diseases, we must heal the gut, manage stress, rule out heavy metal poisoning, rule out infectious causes, include exercise, eliminate inflammatory foods (gluten, grains, legumes), and ensure proper sleep.

Case Study: Debbie

Debbie came to my clinic after having been diagnosed with rheumatoid arthritis (RA) by a rheumatologist. She brought the results of her bloodwork with her, and these confirmed she had an elevated rheumatoid factor (antibody) in her blood as well as symmetrical swelling in her joints, especially her wrists and hands. The specialist had explained that she had a lifelong condition of RA (named it), prescribed three different drugs (tamed it), and given her numerous pamphlets to explain the cause of these symptoms and side effects of the toxic drugs (blamed it).

Debbie was referred to my clinic by a relative I had treated for a similar condition. As I spoke with Debbie, I realized that neither the specialist nor her general practitioner had asked about her psychosocial history or her current circumstances. As it turned out, she and her husband owned a small business that they had successfully expanded over decades. They had worked hard and the business had become lucrative. Three years before Debbie was diagnosed with RA, her son had married and the young couple had come to live in the large farmhouse with Debbie and her husband. After a few months, the daughter-in-law had become confrontational and belligerent to the family, and it was discovered that she had a history of drug and alcohol abuse. She had been doing the family's bookkeeping and banking and had been embezzling thousands of dollars, which had put the family near bankruptcy. When confronted about this, the daughter-in-law had lashed out at Debbie and her husband physically and verbally. A messy divorce ensued, and the former daughter-in-law's lawyers were now fighting for half of the farm that the family had worked so hard to grow. Needless to say, Debbie was understandably anxious and upset by all of these events.

I learned that Debbie's health problems had begun shortly after her son got married. Initially, she had irritable bowel syndrome (page 103) and heartburn and was prescribed a drug called Losec, which she took for one year. Later, she was prescribed strong antibiotics for an *H. pylori* infection (page 102). She wasn't sleeping because her daughter-in-law was very domineering and physically abusive, and Debbie became fearful for herself and her son. Throughout the year before her RA diagnosis, she had complained of joint swelling and fatigue, which is why her general practitioner had finally referred her to a rheumatologist. With this new information, I proceeded to examine Debbie and test her hormone levels. Unsurprisingly, I found high inflammatory markers and elevated cortisol, a stress hormone.

I asked Debbie to wait a few months before filling the prescriptions for the three arthritis drugs the specialist had recommended. Instead, I suggested we try an integrative approach using the REFRAME toolkit (Chapter 9). Firstly, I counseled her extensively about the mind-brain-body connection and explained that she had been in a state of chronic stress for the past three years. I explained how stress was contributing to the issues in her gut, where much of her immune system is located. Once she understood the root of her health issue and was able to connect the dots in the timeline of her health, I taught her how to use the breath, mind, word (BMW) meditation techniques (page 82) on a daily basis. To support the PNS, I put her on the 5R gut program (page 110) to eliminate inflammatory foods, recommended supplements to support her immune system, and got her further counseling to deal with the stressors.

After a few months, Debbie's rheumatoid factor (antibody) count had decreased dramatically. The swelling in her joints had resolved, her gut felt much better, and she was sleeping. By managing her stress and settling her gut issues with the 5R program, we were able to address her autoimmune response with natural and holistic means. She didn't have to suffer the side effects of the arthritis drugs or take these medications for the rest of her life. After the legal dust settled, the divorce was finalized, and the courts ruled in her favor, Debbie was able to regain her health. She was able to keep the farm without the threat of losing it to her former daughter-in-law. Stress had taken a huge toll on her immune system.

Debbie did have to make some drastic shifts in her thinking and her lifestyle, but she has been able to maintain them up to now and has had no further recurrence of rheumatoid arthritis.

➤ Food Allergies

Food sensitivities and food allergies are on the rise. Most of us know at least one person—if not many—who avoid certain foods because eating them causes discomfort. It's important to distinguish between *food sensitivities* (also called intolerances), in which the reaction to a particular food is triggered by the digestive tract, and *food allergies*, in which the reaction is initiated by the immune system. Both occur soon after eating and can cause intensely uncomfortable gas and bloating, diarrhea, and abdominal pain and cramping. Common food sensitivities include intolerances to lactose (dairy), lectins (grains and legumes and fruits in the nightshade family), and gluten (proteins found in wheat, barley, and rye). Sensitivities occur because the body is unable to process the content of the food. People with lactose intolerance lack an enzyme that converts the lactose of milk into sugars the body can digest. This excess of undigested lactose causes the pain and bloating people experience.

In contrast, food allergies occur due to an immune response to an antigen within the food. When immune cells recognize a morsel of food as "foreign," they mount a counterattack, fighting an infection that isn't present. Allergies include nut allergies (such as peanuts) and shellfish allergies (crustaceans and mollusks). In severe anaphylaxis allergies, even a tiny amount of an allergy-causing food can cause severe and sometimes fatal reactions such as hives and swollen airways.

Increased toxins and pollutants in the environment and the food we eat, excessive hygiene, and a rise in caesarean births seem to be some of the reasons why food allergies have become more prevalent and more severe. Reducing stress and repairing the gut with the 5R gut program help to support and strengthen our immune system, eliminating some sensitivities and reducing the severity of allergy symptoms.

HOW TO CULTIVATE A
HEALTHY IMMUNE SYSTEM

Proper gut function is essential for the immune system to flourish and grow. Unlike traditional medical practitioners, doctors of integrative medicine address the role of diet, gut health, and stress to heal the immune system. The aim is to improve and support rather than suppress the immune system, as conventional drug therapies do. Emerging data[7] suggests we need to use therapeutic strategies to treat early symptoms of immune dysfunction and look at the root causes—genetics, environment, and intestinal permeability—in order to prevent and manage more severe immune disorders such as AI diseases. By getting to the root cause of the immune dysfunction, perhaps we can better understand how to strengthen the immune system and manage the painful or debilitating symptoms without harming the rest of the body's systems. Taking care of severe symptoms is essential to quality of life. Drugs have a place—they are helpful in severe cases and can reduce the permanent damage to joints—however, *only* taking care of the symptoms is costly, comes with many side effects, and is not sustainable.

I like to compare AI diseases to a large, deep, dark ditch. Once our immune system has memorized a certain protein pathway, it remains forever in our immune memory. In other words, once you dig that ditch, you can never get rid of it. However, you can walk away from the ditch to avoid falling in. And that's exactly the approach I take to treating AI diseases. Eating a diet high in refined sugar, high-fructose corn syrup, and flour brings you close to the edge of the ditch and often causes flare-ups. Adding poor sleep, lack of exercise, multiple stressors, and alcohol brings you even closer to the ditch, to the point you could even fall in and experience the full-blown effects of the disease. By being impeccable with your diet, managing stress, and getting proper rest, you can stay a long way from that ditch and the symptoms of autoimmune diseases.

Examine Your Immune Environment

The key to a healthy immune system is being aware of the whole body. After all, the primary function of our immune system is to protect our self and ward off nonself, whether those foreign invaders are inside the body or out. Conventional medicine has been very good at treating many diseases, but AI diseases largely remain a mystery to scientists who focus on one part of the system without looking at the bigger picture. What functional medicine teaches us is that an integrated approach to understanding and supporting the body's defense strategies achieves measurable results. In his introductory text, Jorge H. Daruna writes, "Psychoneuroimmunology is the most integrative health science discipline in existence."[8]

Unlike other body systems, to boost and support immunity means drawing on tools for every part of our body: re-setting our ANS through deep, controlled breathing (page 82), upgrading our inner dialogue (page 28), tapping into our conscious brain (page 55), eating a healthy diet (page 110), exercising our muscles (page 143), regulating our heart rate (page 182), and reclaiming our proper rest (page 209). Only by closely examining each of these environments and making positive changes to reduce chronic stress and cultivate a health mindset can we have true immune system health. I refer to this combination of tools as my REFRAME toolkit (more on this in the next chapter).

➤ Follow an Anti-Inflammatory Diet

Immune dysfunction often begins with and is exacerbated by an imbalance in the gut microbiome. An anti-inflammatory diet consists of foods that reduce inflammatory responses and restore beneficial bacteria to the digestive tract. This diet involves replacing red meats and foods made with sugar and refined grains with nutrient-rich plant-based whole foods. Cruciferous vegetables such as broccoli, kale, cabbage, cauliflower, and brussels sprouts are especially beneficial, as are healthy fats from avocados, olive oil, and coconut oil as well as fatty fish (salmon, sardines) and nuts (almonds, unless allergic). Consuming fermented foods rich in probiotic cultures, such as kombucha, sauerkraut, kefir, and homemade unsweetened plain yogurt—all excellent sources of beneficial bacteria—helps to rebuild damaged microflora. Supplements that promote and support the immune system can also help (see Appendix B).

➤ My Story

During the years following my injury, I got recurrent colds in the winter and more allergy symptoms in the spring. Previously I had rarely had the flu, but in those years I was down frequently with severe flu-like illnesses that sometimes required antibiotics. My immune system likely had taken a beating over the years. I didn't make the connections until a blood test revealed a suppressed white blood cell count and elevated C-reactive protein, a nonspecific protein that goes up when the body is inflamed.

After a few years of being ill, my blood tests started to show elevated levels of thyroid antibodies and the endocrinologist wanted me to start on thyroid hormones, as he suspected hypothyroidism. Before going that route, I began to monitor my antibodies and I noticed that whenever I ate poorly and took more pain medications, my gut symptoms got worse and my antibody count would go higher. Based on research I had been doing on inflammation, gut health, and the immune system through the Institute for Functional Medicine, I decided to follow an anti-inflammatory diet that helped to repair my gut, got more sleep, and managed my pain using mindfulness and relaxation techniques, massage, and acupuncture. My antibody count went down.

The same was true of patients in my clinical practice. I observed that their antibody count often fluctuated depending on what was happening with their gut, diet, sleep, and stress levels. All those factors impair the gut's immune system (GALT). I learned a valuable health lesson: all of our body systems are interrelated. If we can support the immune system and gut health, we promote better immunity.

➤ Cultivate Excellent Sleep Habits

Adequate sleep is essential to maintain a strong immune system. Cytokines are cell-signaling molecules that carry information between the immune system and the brain and central nervous system. During the day, when our stress hormones are usually highest, cytokines carry predominantly anti-inflammatory messages, encoding information about new antigens and quickly instructing our immune cells to fight off these foreign invaders. At night, however, cytokines carry pro-inflammatory messages, signaling cells to repair the damage and consolidating the information they've learned about the antigens so they can adapt and be better prepared to fight off subsequent attacks from the same invaders. Slow-wave (NREM stage 3) sleep is especially needed to promote the release of growth hormone and immune-boosting factors and to support this long-lasting "immunological memory" that helps us recall previously encountered antigens and adapt by creating antibodies to fight off future infections.[9]

> ➤ Use Meditation and Relaxation to Manage
>   Stress Effectively

Chronic stress, such as ongoing toxic relationships at home or at work or financial troubles, can take a huge toll on the immune system, because it invokes a persistent pro-inflammatory response, or chronic low-grade inflammation. Managing stress through deep, controlled breathing is the foundation of change, because a clear and focused mind makes good dietary and lifestyle choices and can better regulate the triggers that cause stress hormones to surge and compromise our immune system. Meditation helps us recognize our familiar, often negative thought patterns and realize we have a conscious choice about whether or not to believe them.

Meditation quiets the mind and boosts antibodies, and a daily practice stimulates the immune system and the centers of the brain that control positive emotions, awareness, and anxiety. Researchers have shown that when the brain is in a state of deep relaxation associated with alpha brain waves, fewer excitatory neurons are firing and anxiety is reduced. Instead, the brain releases more endorphins, melatonin, and serotonin, all chemicals associated with calm, tranquility, and pleasure. Patients with AI diseases who meditate regularly and manage their stress—by responding to life's challenges rather than reacting to them—are able to reduce the number of relapses of their disease.[10]

Teams of researchers from both Harvard Medical School and the University of California[11] concluded that turning up the PNS through meditation had measurable effects on our genes and ability to fight infections. They studied the blood of women who attended a meditation retreat and examined nearly 20,000 different genes to determine if there were changes in their gene expression before and after the retreat. All the groups of women experienced a shift in the expression of their genes related to stress, inflammation, and wound healing. The group of experienced meditators had even more remarkable shifts in genes related to fighting viral infections. Interestingly, these women also showed healthier aging.

Scientists have studied this incredible "mind-gene" connection by measuring the length of the telomeres at the ends of our chromosomes. Telomeres are thought to protect our genetic material in a similar way to the little plastic protectors at the ends of shoelaces that stop the laces from fraying. Chronic stress shortens the telomeres, and shorter telomeres are associated with higher rates of disease and shorter lifespan. Changes in our DNA, like shorter telomeres on our chromosomes, can be passed along to the next generation genetically, which may explain why certain AI diseases seem to run in families.

A review article published in the *Annals of the New York Academy of Sciences* summarized the scientific findings on meditation from a number of renowned universities and institutions.[12] C-reactive protein, an inflammatory marker, was repeatedly reduced through meditation alone. Furthermore, individuals with human immunodeficiency virus (HIV) who meditated underwent a positive and protective increase in T-cell activity, which helps the body fight off nasty opportunistic infections.

Rudolph Tanzi from Harvard University and the Massachusetts General Hospital said, "Meditation is one of the ways to engage in restorative activities that may provide relief for our immune systems, easing the day-to-day stress of a body constantly trying to protect itself."[13] More studies are underway, but there is still a lot of work to do to understand the full impact of our state of mind on our immune system and genes.

➤ Exercise Regularly

While extreme exercise can be harmful to the immune system, we know that moderate movement helps support immunity and is a big benefit. Just thirty to sixty minutes of walking, swimming, or cycling three times a week in patients with rheumatoid arthritis reduces disease activity, improves cardiac fitness, and more importantly improves immune function.[14] This means reduced infection and less inflammation. Harmful immune cells (cytotoxic T cells) are less active after bouts of exercise.

➤ Adopt an Attitude of Gratitude and Positivity

Gratitude is key to recovering the immune system as it rewires our brain to the positive and makes a neural shift in the brain chemicals for health. Cultivating gratitude transforms the brain at a molecular level. With functional magnetic resonance imaging (fMRI), people who practice gratitude on a regular basis have been shown to elicit a higher production of dopamine, thereby improving neuronal function.[15] Numerous studies show that gratitude as a daily practice helps people find meaning, purpose, greater compassion, self-acceptance, and better relationships with others. It makes us less reactive and less prone to cortisol surges. Grateful people sleep better and report less anxiety and depression.

Listen to your inner dialogue and notice your thought patterns. Is your mind focused on what is missing or on being grateful for what is present? Make a conscious shift by keeping a daily gratitude journal. Better sleep, improved mood, and a stronger immune system are compelling reasons to be grateful!

Research has shown that we perform better at our work and in our relationships when we are happier.[16] If our brain is wired for happiness, we make better chemicals that support the immune system. Happy people don't necessarily experience happier life events, they just look for the small positives daily! Mel Robbins talks about the three S's, which are story, savor, and smile (page 56). Taking the time to change your story, savor the good stuff, and smile triggers happy hormones, lowers anxiety, and reduces stress, which improves immune function.

The Benefits of a Healthy Immune System

It is easy to take a healthy immune system for granted. Most of us walk around breathing freely through our noses all day, never considering this complex system until we catch a cold or a flu and that nasal patency is gone. Then we weep and moan as we fill a steady stream of tissues with mucus and sputum and wonder how to repair our broken immune system.

A robust ability to fight off infections, large and small, allows us to exist in our germ-infested world: shaking hands, boarding planes, using restrooms, and visiting our loved ones in the hospital. Although we don't yet know how to prevent AI diseases, I believe that diet, healthy lifestyle, and proper stress management can slow down or stop an AI disease in its very early stages of development.

CONCLUSION

Today our immune system rarely gets downtime and we suffer more inflammation. While temporary inflammation helps us heal, chronic inflammation does not. And stress-related chronic inflammation increasingly shows up as painful food allergies and autoimmune diseases.

Chronic stress compromises our immune system, and a vicious cycle can develop as our impaired immune system causes us additional physical and psychological stress. However, our immune system continues to develop and learn new ways to defend our body. I expect that more research in this area of stress and adaptive immunity will help us understand this cycle better and find solutions.

Meditation improves our ability to fight infections, and other similar mind-based tools will likely prove effective. So tapping into our mind and using it to alter our immune system function is a powerful way to improve our health. Where conventional medicine has traditionally looked at each symptom and prescribed a solution, integrative medicine gives us a whole new way of looking at the disease. Our bodies are interconnected networks. When our mind, brain, and body are in balance, good health follows. When one or more are out of balance, ill health is the result. What I offer you, then, is a toolkit of solutions.

Illness in one part of the body affects the body as a whole, and it's important to find the root cause. If that root cause is chronic stress, any of the seven tools in the REFRAME toolkit (Chapter 9) will help. Are you experiencing hypertension? Consistent nights of good-quality sleep will help. Are you depressed? Thirty minutes of regular movement will make a difference.

Are you suffering from irritable bowel syndrome? Cultivating a health mindset will help. And all of these tools will help boost your immune system and keep it in fighting form.

9.

The REFRAME Toolkit:

Seven Tools to Re-set Your Health

TO BE OPTIMALLY healthy, heal pain, and control anxiety and fatigue, we must learn to manage chronic stress. The REFRAME toolkit is a program I developed for myself and my patients to help connect the dots between physical symptoms and our mental and emotional state, integrate the body systems, and create optimal health using mind-brain-body principles. REFRAME stands for *Re-*set, *E*xercise, *F*ood, *R*est, *A*ssess, *M*indset, and *E*xamine, and these are the key areas I use to assess and treat patients in my clinical practice. These key words address each of the areas of the body we've seen in the previous chapters.

I particularly like the acronym REFRAME because psychologists talk about "cognitive reframing," which means voluntarily looking at ideas, events, beliefs, and emotions in our lives and trying to find more positive alternatives that serve us better. This concept has become popular among business managers making changes within organizations too. When they meet resistance from people who want to maintain the status quo, they encourage those employees to reflect on the benefits of the change rather than the drawbacks.

In the context of the body, assessing our inner dialogue and shifting our point of reference from a negative, illness mindset to a positive, health mindset—reframing it—allows the autonomic nervous system (ANS) to work for us, not against us. That is, instead of reacting to automatic thoughts, which keeps us in fight-or-flight mode, we can respond mindfully to conscious ones, which allows us to spend more time in rest-and-digest mode and achieve better outcomes for our health. The result is less exposure to the harmful effects of stress hormones at a cellular level to optimize health.

The tools in the REFRAME kit are designed to help us apply the brakes and take control of chronic stress. I recommend that no matter what your symptoms, you begin with the re-set tool. The short-term benefits of re-setting the ANS through controlled breathing and mindful meditation are immediately obvious because we feel more calm, rational, and energized. The long-term benefits of managing the ANS and chronic stress through controlled breathing as well as exercise, food, rest, and other tools are less obvious but even more powerful for our body. They include a lower risk of heart disease, improved immune function, better gut function, restful sleep, and happier mood, just to name a few. And cultivating a health mindset in any part of the body brings a multitude of benefits to the whole: we have fewer health issues, we begin to recognize where we might go off course, and we know how to get back on track if we do.

Life will always present challenges, but by recognizing chronic stress and its symptoms and knowing how to control it by using a variety of tools to regulate our ANS, we become healthier and enjoy life more. Everyone is different when it comes to finding the actions that work best. Experiment. Find out which tools help you the most. And keep believing you have power over your health. Remember, the mind is the most powerful tool we have to regulate stress. Mastering your mind to control your ANS is ultimately taking the power of your health into your own hands, making you your own best doctor! Read on to discover more about each tool.

1. RE-SET

Re-set refers to our ability to stop, recognize that we are in a state of stress, and take steps to regulate our ANS. We know that both overt and covert stress cause many of us to lead our lives with the sympathetic nervous system (SNS)—the gas—turned up too high much of the time, and that our body systems become inflamed and ill as a result. There is an alternative. We can move through our days feeling calm and responding to what life brings us based on new wisdom and thought processes. We need to turn on our parasympathetic nervous system (PNS)—our brakes—to do that.

I find the combination of controlled breathing inspired by Dr. Herbert Benson's Relaxation Response and mindful meditation inspired by Jon Kabat-Zinn to be highly effective. I call the technique I use my breath, mind, word (BMW) meditation. It encompasses breathing and muscle relaxation techniques that turn on the vagus nerve, causing the ANS to slow down, as well as meditation techniques that focus attention on the present moment to turn off the inner dialogue and incessant chatter and allow slower, more reflective thoughts. Repeating a word also helps to slow down brain activity and focus my attention. These three steps together get you to that "sweet spot" where you feel your body and mind shift to a calmer, more relaxed state.

BMW Meditation

BMW meditation means engaging the breath (to relax the muscles of the diaphragm and the body), the mind (to be consciously present), and the word (to entrain the brain). This meditation can be done anywhere, anytime, but I suggest you start with ten minutes of BMW meditation in the morning and ten minutes in the evening before you go to bed. I also like to do forty-five- to sixty-second mini meditations to re-set my ANS throughout the day when I face the most stressors. You can even do a walking meditation.

1. Inhale deeply through the nose, using your diaphragm to take breaths that reach right down to your belly. Count to five as you inhale.

2. Exhale through the mouth, making the exhale longer than the inhale.

3. After about two minutes, relax your muscles from your head to your toes as you exhale.

4. Bring your attention to your breath as you continue to inhale and exhale slowly and deeply. Simply observe your breath.

5. As you exhale, begin to silently say a word such as peace, amen, home, or om.

6. Continue inhaling and exhaling slowly and deeply for ten to twelve minutes. If your mind wanders, gently bring it back to the present by focusing on your breath and your word. The key is to be mindful of your thoughts, stay in the present moment, and become the observer of your thoughts while doing the breathing and muscle relaxation.

Everyone manages stress differently, but the best advice I can give you is *to actually do it*. Perhaps in the future an app will re-set our ANS with just the press of a button! Now, however, meditation is the first step to making big changes in your life, because it helps you become aware of your thoughts and consciously choose your mindset. Add controlled breathing, which turns off the stress hormones and manufactures chemicals of healing, and you are well on your way to making choices that support your health. Adapt the BMW meditation or other breathing and meditation techniques to suit your own life and keep it simple. Remember, the best plan is the one you will actually follow—even, or especially, on the hardest days.

The re-set tool helps you to be present, be aware of your thoughts, and observe them without reacting so you can choose how to respond. A focused, clear mind makes good dietary and lifestyle choices and can better regulate the triggers that cause stress hormones to surge.

2. EXERCISE

I dedicated an entire chapter to movement because motion is lotion! The bottom line is to move as much as possible for as many years as possible. Being still for too long makes us sick and stiff because the body needs oxygen, and exercise helps circulate oxygenated blood throughout the body. Exercise is beneficial for a healthy heart, brain, immune system, and so much more. Exercise helps the body to integrate all the systems and create resilience to stress. It is also the best way to burn off excess adrenaline and cortisol.

Remember that there are three types of exercise and you want to do two types each day.

- *Cardio.* We need at least thirty to forty-five minutes of exercise a day with our heart rate over 120 beats per minute.

- *Strength training.* Our body needs mechanical stress to build strength, and weights are a great way to do this. Aim for two fifteen-minute sessions a week, starting with five pounds and gradually increasing to twelve to fifteen pounds.

- *Stretching.* Make it a habit to stretch for a couple of minutes when you wake up and also intermittently at your desk at work to prevent tight muscle spasm. Yoga or Pilates is a great way for your body to integrate the muscles, bones, and fascia to prevent stiffness.

All of our tissues need different exercises to thrive. Each of the muscles in our body gets used to particular exercises, so cross-train (change up the sports and the movements you do) for optimal health. Use the Smart, Motivation, Urgency, Focus, Leverage, and Decisions (SMUFLD) formula (page 145) to help you make changes to your lifestyle, specifically developing a healthier diet and a more active lifestyle. This formula gives you the tools and motivation to start now, start small, and build up. Step by step and with a bit of effort, develop and maintain an exercise mindset and achieve great gains for your health.

3. FOOD

Food is fuel, but that doesn't mean we can eat whatever we want whenever we want. In fact, how we digest our food is as important as what food we eat. Many of us eat to soothe our emotions and then feel anger, shame, or guilt about it, which results in painful and embarrassing gut issues. Being mindful about what we eat, when we eat it, and most importantly, how we feel when we eat, are the keys to optimal digestion, nutrient absorption, and better health.

· Choose healthy foods rich in vegetables, fiber, good fats (for example, nuts, seeds, avocados), and healthy proteins (for example, free-range meats). Limit salt and alcohol.

· Eat purposefully. Taking time to chew and taste your food engages the vagus nerve and the PNS. When the nervous system works for us, not against us, it absorbs more nutrients and helps the body heal and repair.

· Consume fermented foods, such as sauerkraut, kombucha, and natural unsweetened yogurt to keep your gut flora and microbiome healthy.

· Avoid refined sugar, flour, and processed meats (and other processed foods), which cause inflammation in the gut. Remember, the gut makes 80 to 85 percent of our serotonin. When we are happy, our gut knows it!

· Ask your health practitioner about supplements. Many people don't get enough vitamin D, magnesium, or omega-3 fatty acids in their diet. Vegans may need vitamin B12 supplements, iron, or certain amino acids.

Re-set your mindset for health when you sit down to eat. And if chronic stress has already affected your digestion, make better food choices and ease gut issues using the 5R gut program (page 110).

· *Remove* the foods that irritate the gut.

· *Replace* any secretions or enzymes missing from the gut.

· *Repair* the gut by eating plant-based whole foods and clean fats (add supplements, if needed).

· *Repopulate* the healthy bacteria in the gut with prebiotic and probiotic foods.

· *Relax/rest* the mind and the gut to optimize digestion and nutrient absorption.

4. REST

Downtime and sleep are vital to our well-being because it's mostly when we rest that the body manufactures important hormones that help to heal and repair our cells and tissues. This downtime also allows the brain to "unplug." In our busy lives, many of us rely on "survival" brain. We react to situations, and our fight-or-flight reaction releases stress hormones. When we rest and give our brain time to be creative and contemplative, we release chemicals that help us feel happier, and we respond to situations by making conscious decisions. Try one or more of these tips to get high-quality rest and a good night's sleep:

· Use relaxation and visualization techniques to regulate your breathing, engage your conscious mind, and calm your nervous system.

- Meditate, engage in contemplative prayer or other spiritual or religious practices, or do any activity where you find peace.

- Unplug from technology. Set aside time in the day when you are not "connected" to a computer, phone, or any other device.

- Devise a personal sleep routine. Include rituals that create a feeling of calm, train your body to expect them, and aim for six to eight hours of good-quality sleep every night.

- If needed, speak to your health practitioner about strategies to deal with insomnia, such as sleep hypnosis, natural supplements, or cognitive behavioral therapy.

Observe your beliefs about sleep. Do you consider it a badge of honor to get by on very little sleep? It's time to change that belief! Use positive self-talk, set up boundaries with yourself and others, and think about how much better you'll feel when you're more rested. Science shows that a rested brain and body are more productive and make better decisions.

5. ASSESS

Being healthy takes time and effort! We are at our healthiest when our physical, mental, and emotional health are all in balance. And just as we set work goals, finance goals, or relationship goals, we can set health goals. Remember, we are a key player in our own health. The more we know about our health and what we want to achieve, the better we can work toward it and enlist the help of others to support us. Regular assessments are a great way to become aware of our health needs, set realistic goals, evaluate our progress, and celebrate our successes along the way.

No matter where you are in your health journey, it's important to focus on the journey itself rather than worrying about meeting those goals. After all, getting healthy is best when you enjoy the journey.

· To begin, ask your health-care practitioner for a whole-body health assessment or use the self-assessment questions at the start of each chapter in this book. Use the results to pinpoint areas of your health that could benefit from attention.

· With your health-care practitioner, set some realistic health goals. If it's a big goal, break it down into smaller, achievable goals.

· Evaluate your progress regularly by doing self-assessments. Are you on track? How are your actions affecting other areas of your health? Do you need to change one or more of your goals? Have you achieved any of your health goals? Is it time to set new ones?

· Make time to celebrate your successes. If you encounter a setback, be gentle with yourself. With your health-care practitioner, assess your existing goals, recommit to them or change them as needed.

It's important to know what your health needs are and which areas might need more attention. Exercise, sleep, peace of mind, or diet? Assessments help to make sure you address the basic pillars of health.

6. MINDSET

Mindset matters! Again and again in this book, I've highlighted that a health mindset is the key to a healthy body. But most people are not born with a health mindset. They have cultivated it over time by taking action every day toward a health goal, even if they do it because it's good for them and not because they love it. Those habits eventually become automatic—going to the gym every day, eating vegetables at every meal, going to bed at 9 p.m. just become part of their routine.

Check your inner dialogue. Do you have an illness mindset? Are your automatic negative thoughts sabotaging your ability to heal? If so, re-set your mindset. Be sure your mind is calm and quiet, and then use the stop, observe, detach, affirm (SODA) technique:

- *Stop* and gain control over your thoughts. Be the mind that does the thinking.

- *Observe* your mind witnessing your thoughts and emotions without judgment or action.

- *Detach* from negative, automatic fear-based pathways once you recognize them.

- *Affirm* another, positive thought to replace the automatic negative thought.

To develop a healthy mindset, you need to remain open and curious. Challenge your automatic behaviors, thoughts, and beliefs. Critically assess your inner dialogue about the choices you make. Create a clear, conscious mindset for self-care, so you will have better boundaries with work, relationships, food, exercise, and alcohol. Cultivate a deep knowing that you hold some control over what happens to your body and, most importantly, that you control how you respond to a situation.

Cultivating a health mindset and achieving your health goals is much easier when you

· are inspired to change,

· are persistent,

· find your passion,

· practice self-compassion and kindness,

· find something or someone to be grateful for,

· believe in yourself, your goal, and your ability to achieve it, and

· practice patience, letting go, and non-judgment.

As you are shifting your mindset, imagine your story of success, savor the gains, and smile to feel positive about the changes. As you train your brain to a new outlook, repeat statements such as, "I haven't mastered a health mindset *yet*" to make a stronger connection to the positive and give yourself room to grow.

7. EXAMINE

This book is designed to empower you to become more mind and body aware and to know when to seek help. It is not a substitute for your health-care provider. Stress hormones are the root cause of many illnesses and diseases, but genetics, injuries, infections, and toxins can play a part. Trained professionals can often spot the physical signs of disease before you catch them in a self-assessment. They can order diagnostic tests to confirm or rule out a suspected illness. They can recommend evidence-based interventions to create excellent health. If you have persistent symptoms, make an appointment for a physical examination and please ensure you get the proper care and treatment from your health-care practitioner.

Taking responsibility for your beliefs, thoughts, choices, and behaviors and asking the right questions helps your health-care provider to help you. For example, know your personal risks for disease. If you smoke or consume alcohol, other substances, or food to cope with pain or stress, your health-care practitioner may be able to help you quit. Be proactive and advocate for your health. For example, if needed, ask your health-care provider to monitor your blood pressure, cholesterol, and blood sugar levels.

Ideally, practice prevention so you need less intervention. Apply the principles of mind-body medicine no matter how serious your health challenges. For example, a health mindset is beneficial whether you feel anxious before an exam or a chemotherapy treatment. Many cancer treatment centers are adding integrative medicine and mindfulness-based stress reduction techniques to their regular treatment plans. These are safe because there are no drug interactions with mind-body medicine!

How the REFRAME Toolkit Can Help

We know that pain, anxiety, fatigue, insomnia, and gut problems are just a few of the symptoms of chronic stress. If you experience these symptoms, doing a BMW meditation every day to re-set your ANS is a good place to start. You will likely become more energized and more resilient to the effects of stress and disease. More importantly, learning to master your mind and calm your nervous system gives you the ability to make conscious choices about your health. You become an active participant in choosing health every day, from what you eat to how active you are to how long and how deeply you sleep. The more integrated and collaborative your mind and body are, the better your chances of living a long and healthy life.

We know that sickness and dysfunction in one body system affects all the others, which is why "connecting the dots" to get to the root cause is so important. The REFRAME toolkit addresses mental, physical, and emotional symptoms. And while medical interventions can help in some situations, knowing how to manage your emotional health to prevent disease is your responsibility. You know your mind the best, you know what your stressors are, and you now understand how your emotional stress can rev up your ANS and manifest as physical symptoms in your body.

As a patient after my car accident, I found that mind-body integration was the key to my own healing. And as a physician, I see how mind-body integration makes a difference to the health outcomes of my patients. Learning to regulate our neurobiological system is the key to resolving many of our long-term health problems. My sincere wish is to educate and inspire as many people as possible to take control of their autonomic nervous system. Most people can cultivate a positive, health mindset once they decide to, and that simple decision is not only affordable and can be done at any time by anyone, it is also highly effective.

I truly believe that people who embrace a health mindset and work to develop that mindset are doing a remarkable service to themselves, their health-care providers, and their communities. So cultivate your health mindset and use these practical tools to be your healthiest self!

Acknowledgments

HAVING AN IDEA and turning it into a book is a daunting task filled with trials and tribulations. Many people helped me make this book happen, and I could not have done it without them. I am truly grateful and blessed.

I want to sincerely thank my husband, who has been a constant source of patience, support, and inspiration as I've navigated the writing and publishing world. He has stood by me as I typed into the wee hours of the morning, quietly bringing me ginger tea without breaking my focus. His unwavering faith in my ability to get my message out to the world has motivated me to keep going. My son, Shaan, is an emergency physician and sees very sick patients. He and I have had very interesting discussions about prevention and intervention models of medicine and learned a lot from each other. Ultimately, both medical models are essential in health care and not mutually exclusive. My daughter, Shalni, meticulously combed through the initial chapters for grammar and syntax, and I thank her for her beautiful presence. I am so thankful for my loving sister, Joty Manocha, who has been my biggest fan and cheerleader on this project. I love and appreciate all of you, especially when you have expressed understanding during the last two years when I took time away from being with you.

I want to acknowledge my dear friend and "soul sister" who has walked on this journey with me since we met twenty years ago. Dr. Nishi Dhawan and I co-founded the Westcoast Women's Clinic. She was the wind beneath my sails, and I am grateful for her encouragement to write this book. To have a like-minded physician's support while facing the challenges and rewards of practicing integrative medicine was immense. I would not have had the courage or strength to forge this path without Nishi by my side. Dr. Jeanny Wong, my general practitioner and friend since our internship, was instrumental in my physical recovery after my accident. She guided me during all the medical interventions that were needed and supported me as I began to explore integrative medicine as a way to further heal myself.

My patients have taught me so much, allowing me into their lives to walk in their shoes as I continue to grow and learn from them. Our patient-doctor partnership benefits from our openness, curiosity, and connection. I am extremely grateful for their trust, confidence, and courage to transform their lives using principles of integrative medicine. My friend Michael Bentley coached me to share my personal story as a patient and the reason why I am so passionate about the importance of mind-brain-body connections. Without his encouragement, this would have been simply a medical book. He checked in with me regularly to keep me on track. I am grateful for his guidance and wisdom.

The biggest thank you to Rob Sanders and his team at Greystone for having confidence in me as a first-time writer and recognizing the importance of bringing the message of self-care to the masses. I am eternally grateful to Lucy Kenward, for her extreme diligence, research, and impeccable attention to detail to help me stay on track and express very difficult concepts in an easy-to-understand manner. She is principled, works with integrity and passion on a project, and is willing to go the extra mile to support and guide an author. I genuinely appreciate her efforts to organize and galvanize my work.

Alison Caldwell was a great writing coach and got me in the habit of writing regularly as I started this book. Words cannot express (an irony for a writer) my heartfelt thanks to Melody Owen, who was an amazing source of expertise and took me to the next level in prepping my manuscript for the publisher. She worked tirelessly to provide structure and clarity for my message.

I was fortunate to have students help me with some research. In particular, Dylan Suyama was extremely skilled and diligent at finding relevant studies. His writing potential is immense. Remi Kandal was very helpful for the Brain chapter of this book. Dr. Shannon Trainor and Sharon Pendlington, thank you for your patient proofreading. Sharon's knowledge and passion for holistic nutrition was so helpful. And thank you to Dr. Rob Comey for help with the Sleep chapter and to Dr. Shirin Kalyan for help with the Immune chapter. Also, thanks to Dr. Leora Kuttner and Dr. Bianca Rucker for their guidance.

Appendix A:
Gut Health Assessment

This questionnaire is designed to give your doctor insight into how your intestinal system is functioning. Please circle the number that most accurately describes your current lifestyle, and then tally the total number in each subsection.

Please indicate if you use any of the following medications and how often	Rare	Occasional	Often	Frequent
Antacids	0	1	4	8
Laxatives	0	1	4	8
Antibiotics	0	1	4	8
Oral antifungals	0	1	4	8
Acid inhibitors (e.g., Zantac, Losec, Tecta)	0	1	4	8
Acetaminophen (e.g., Tylenol)	0	1	4	8
Anti-inflammatory meds (e.g., ibuprofen, aspirin)	0	1	4	8

How many times do you consume the following foods in 1 week?	0–1	2–4	5–9	10+
Sugary treats	0	1	4	8
Soft drinks	0	1	4	8
Coffee or black tea	0	1	4	8
Fried foods	0	1	4	8
Spicy foods	0	1	4	8

Section A	Rare	Occasional	Often	Frequent
1. Indigestion: food sits in stomach for a long time after eating	0	1	4	8
2. Excessive burping, belching, or bloating after meals	0	1	4	8
3. Stomach spasms and cramping during or after eating	0	1	4	8
4. Feeling that food sits in your stomach creating uncomfortable fullness and bloating during or after a meal	0	1	4	8
5. Bad taste in your mouth	0	1	4	8
6. Small amounts of food fill you up immediately	0	1	4	8
7. Skip meals or eat erratically because you have no appetite	0	1	4	8
Total				

Section B	Rare	Occasional	Often	Frequent
1. The thought or smell of food aggravates your stomach	0	1	4	8
2. Feel hungry an hour or two after a good-sized meal	0	1	4	8
3. Stomach pain, burning, and/or aching over a period of 1–4 hours after eating	0	1	4	8
4. Stomach pain, burning, and/or aching relieved by eating food, drinking carbonated beverages, cream or milk, or taking antacids	0	1	4	8
5. Burning sensation in the lower part of your chest, especially when lying down or bending forward	0	1	4	8
6. Digestive problems that subside with rest and relaxation	0	1	4	8
7. Burning or aching when eating spicy and fried foods, chocolate, coffee, alcohol, citrus or hot peppers	0	1	4	8
8. Feel a sense of nausea when you eat	0	1	4	8
9. Difficulty or pain when swallowing food or beverages	0	1	4	8
Total				

Section C	Rare	Occasional	Often	Frequent
1. When massaging under your rib cage on your left side, there is pain, tenderness, or soreness	0	1	4	8
2. Indigestion, fullness, or tension in your abdomen is delayed, occurring 2–4 hours after eating a meal	0	1	4	8
3. Lower abdominal discomfort is relieved with the passage of gas or with a bowel movement	0	1	4	8
4. Specific foods or beverages aggravate indigestion	0	1	4	8
5. The consistency or form of your stool changes (e.g., from formed to loose) within the course of a day	0	1	4	8
6. Stool odor is embarrassing	0	1	4	8
7. Undigested food is present in your stool	0	1	4	8
8. Three or more unformed bowel movements daily	0	1	4	8
9. Diarrhea (frequent loose, watery stool)	0	1	4	8
10. Bowel movement shortly after eating (within 30 minutes)	0	1	4	8
Total				

Section D	Rare	Occasional	Often	Frequent
1. Discomfort, pain, or cramps in your lower abdomen	0	1	4	8
2. Emotional stress and/or eating raw fruits and vegetables causes bloating, pain, cramps, or gas	0	1	4	8
3. Necessity to strain during bowel movements	0	1	4	8
4. Stool is small, hard, and dry	0	1	4	8
5. Pass mucus in your stool	0	1	4	8
6. Alternate between constipation and diarrhea	0	1	4	8
7. Rectal pain, itching, or cramping	0	1	4	8
8. Lack of urge to have a bowel movement	0	1	4	8
9. An almost continual need to have a bowel movement	0	1	4	8
Total				

Appendix B:
Supplements

D IETARY SUPPLEMENTS CAN be controversial, and most physicians counsel patients that they don't need supplements unless they have documented deficiencies. Furthermore, supplements are certainly not meant as a substitute for a proper diet, but they provide adjuvant essential nutrients that may be low or missing, so it is very important to speak with your health-care provider to see what is right for you. The reality is that both chronic stress and poor diet contribute to poor absorption in the gut and depletion of micronutrients. Specialized diets, diseases, and medications may also disadvantage your body. Under these circumstances, supplements can be beneficial.

I recommend that everyone eat a diverse, largely plant-based diet rich in tree nuts, seeds, fiber, and good sources of protein (free-range chicken, wild salmon, grass-fed beef). Good fats such as avocados and nut butter, extra-virgin olive oil, and moderate amounts of coconut oil are also recommended. Green leafy vegetables and seaweed (such as nori) are good for phytonutrients, and fiber is prebiotic (helps good bacteria). Fermented foods are essential for maintaining your gut microbiome and providing a ready source of good bacteria.

However, after assessing an individual's health, diet, and lifestyle, I find that some patients benefit from supplements until they can regain their health or make up the deficits. Vegetarians and vegans may require micronutrients such as vitamin B12, iron, or certain amino acids found only in animal products. Our vegetables are grown in soils that are no longer as rich in vitamins and minerals as they once were, and I am seeing an increase in vitamin and mineral deficiencies in some patients.[1] Chronic stress causes a general depletion of vitamins B5, B3, B6, B12, and B1 and minerals such as magnesium. Acid-suppressing drugs and diabetic medications deplete vitamins and minerals as well.

I also recommend supplements when alleviating the symptoms of chronic stress or anxiety requires more than diet and stress management alone. For anxiety, supplements can help calm the autonomic nervous system (ANS) so that medications become more effective. For insomnia, supplements can help regulate sleep enough to relieve the exhaustion that can impede cognitive changes. Certain vitamins and minerals and specific foods help the body heal and recover from stress, and some are great for overall health maintenance. I also address special supplements for sleep, anxiety, gut, and immune system issues.

The supplements listed below are the ones I use most often in my practice; it is certainly not a comprehensive list. Before taking supplements, check with your health-care practitioner about dosage, interactions, and any other safety considerations specific to you. Each product may vary in potency so dosage will depend on the individual company. There is a wider margin of safety with water-soluble vitamins because they are not stored in the body like fat-soluble vitamins. Therefore, proceed with caution when taking high doses of fat-soluble vitamins for a prolonged period of time.

WATER-SOLUBLE VITAMINS

High-potency B complex. These key vitamins, which include B1, B5, B6, and B12, can be depleted by stress. B vitamins maintain the body on many levels. Many of them are involved in nerve and blood cell function. They help with metabolism of food to energy and are essential in almost every biological system in the body, especially skin and brain health.

B12 is especially important to supplement for strict vegetarians, the elderly, those on certain medications (for example, metformin), and people with inflammatory bowel disease (Crohn's disease). Most B vitamins are found naturally in whole grains (brown rice, barley, millet), legumes (beans, lentils), seeds and nuts (sunflower seeds, almonds, walnuts), and dark leafy vegetables (kale, spinach, broccoli). Vitamin B12 is found in the highest quantity in animal products (meat, poultry, fish, and eggs).

Vitamin C. This vitamin helps immune cells such as T cells do their job better and promotes the synthesis of collagen. We cannot say there is robust scientific evidence for taking vitamin C in high doses to prevent a cold, but many people claim it helps. We do know that people deficient in vitamin C have reduced resistance against disease and can become ill when there is a deficiency.

FAT-SOLUBLE VITAMINS

Vitamin D (cholecalciferol, D3). The body can make this vitamin from sunlight or access it through food such as dairy products that have been fortified with vitamin D. Vitamin D supplements are recommended for bone strength and to support mood and immune function. Vitamin D deficiency puts us at higher risk for fractures, autoimmune diseases, and infections. This vitamin is generally deficient for most people who live in temperate climates with little exposure to sunlight on their skin. Many countries have supplemented dairy milk with vitamin D; however, the doses are fairly conservative and only enough to prevent a childhood bone disease called rickets.

Vitamin A. This vitamin occurs naturally in two forms. Preformed vitamin A is found in meats (especially organ meats), fish, poultry, and dairy products. Provitamin A is found in fruits, vegetables, and nuts and is most commonly known as beta-carotene. Both forms are stored in our liver. Vitamin A helps our vision, reproduction, lungs, kidneys, skin, and immune system and contributes to normal growth and development. Some people recommend high doses of Vitamin A to treat adrenal insufficiency, but this approach should be done under the care of a health professional only.

Vitamin E (tocopherols). This antioxidant helps cells to repair DNA and is important for skin and overall immune health. It is found in vegetables, vegetable oils, avocados, squash, seeds, meats, and eggs. Eating foods rich in this vitamin provides enough vitamin E for most people, but those with liver, pancreatic, or Crohn's disease may poorly absorb this vitamin and require extra supplementation. Supplements of vitamin E can also help in times of physical stress, when healing from surgery or burns, or to alleviate a rare deficiency that can cause nerve problems.

We do need certain amounts of fat-soluble vitamins to protect us from deficiency. Since these vitamins are stored in the body, consult your health-care provider before taking supplements. Taking too many fat-soluble vitamins can result in other health problems.

MINERALS

Trace minerals such as calcium, potassium, phosphorus, magnesium, iron, silicon, manganese, barium, copper, and zinc can be found together in a product called SierraSil that I have safely used with my patients. However, I generally avoid single mineral supplements except for magnesium, selenium, and zinc.

Magnesium glycinate or biglycinate. This mineral is helpful for improving sleep, mood, and many enzymes in the body.

Selenium. This mineral is important for thyroid hormones, cognitive function, and fertility. It is found in high concentrations in Brazil nuts—eating two to three of these nuts per day is enough to provide your daily intake.

Zinc. This mineral is found in all of our cells. It is important for wound healing, immune function, and DNA repair and has a healing effect on the gut lining. It is found in nuts, seeds, and animal protein.

SUPPLEMENTS FOR SLEEP

For severe sleep disruption, sometimes one supplement or a combination of supplements may be necessary to induce a normal sleep pattern. Consult with your health-care provider.

Magnesium glycinate. Magnesium is combined with glycine to make it easier to absorb. Dose: Take 200 to 600 mg at bedtime.

Melatonin. This hormone can be taken orally or under the tongue and is helpful for sleep and also as an antioxidant. Dose: Take 3 to 5 mg orally three to four hours before bedtime.

Passion flower. Passion flower increases the levels of gamma-aminobutyric acid (GABA) in the brain, which has a calming effect and may help to treat insomnia, anxiety, and pain. Dose: 200 to 500 mg depending on purity of the product.

Phosphatidylserine. This phospholipid lowers cortisol in the body, improves memory, and helps induce sleep. Dose: Take 100 mg at bedtime. See also the entry for phosphatidylserine in the next section, Supplements for Anxiety.

Valerian root. This root has been used for thousands of years to promote calmness and sleep. Dose: Begin with 400 mg up to two hours before bed. Increase up to 900 mg, if required.

SUPPLEMENTS FOR ANXIETY

Adaptogenic herbs. These healing plants help to calm the nervous system and balance, restore, and protect the body.

Adaptogenic supplements include ashwaganda, rhodiola (Arctic root), holy basil, and a blend of botanicals called Relora. Dose: Consult your health-care practitioner.

Cortisol Manager. This supplement is a mix of stress-reducing ingredients and botanicals that helps to re-establish normal cortisol patterns by regulating the hypothalamic-pituitary axis (HPA). Dose: Take 1 to 2 capsules at bedtime, if you experience early morning wakings or anxiety at night.

L-theanine. This amino acid is found in tea. It induces relaxation without making you drowsy or impairing your heart. Many students find it helpful around exam time to improve memory and concentration and lower stress. The dose depends on the manufactured strengths available.

Phosphatidylserine is a fatty substance that covers and protects the cells in your brain and carries messages between them. It can be found in a cream, AdrenaCalm, or in tablet form. The dose depends on the manufactured strengths available. See also the entry for phosphatidylserine in the previous section, Supplements for Sleep.

SUPPLEMENTS FOR THE GUT

In functional medicine, treating the gut is at the very core of health, as it is responsible for many body systems.

Betaine hydrochloride. This supplement promotes optimal acid pH in the stomach for ideal protein digestion and mineral and vitamin absorption. To determine if you need to take betaine hydrochloride, take 650 mg about one-third of the way into your dinner. If you experience immediate heartburn, your body is producing enough hydrochloric acid. If you do not experience this heartburn, you may benefit from taking betaine hydrochloride on regular basis. Dose: Consult your health-care provider.

Digestive enzymes. Both gut and pancreatic enzymes are helpful for digesting particular foods. As people age, their ability to digest legumes, fiber, and fat diminishes as the enzymes decline. Symptoms of a deficiency include bloating, gas, and flatulence.

L-glutamine. This amino acid repairs damage to the gut and restores the lining. It is fundamental to the digestive and immune systems. It must be used under medical supervision as it can cause brain excitation in some patients. Dose: Take 3,000 to 5,000 mg per day.

Prebiotics. Prebiotics are indigestible fiber, which help good bacteria to survive and multiply. Food sources include garlic, asparagus, artichokes, leeks, dandelion greens, miso, and potato starch. Scientists refer to prebiotics as inulin and oligofructose and note that our diets have dramatically decreased in fiber in the last few decades. There is no formal consensus on the dose, so follow general guidelines. Dose: Take 25 to 40 g of fiber per day.

Probiotics. Human multistrain flora are used to repopulate the gut microbiome when beneficial bacteria have been disrupted or depleted by infection, travel, medication, or chronic stress and eating fermented foods is not enough. Dose: Take a concentrated 25 billion to 100 billion units per day unless you are actively inflamed. Check the exact amount with your health-care provider.

Slippery elm. This supplement, made from the inner bark of the slippery elm tree, has been used for decades to stimulate the production of mucus in the gut. Mucus protects the gut lining from acids, which cause ulcers and inflammation. Dose: Depends on whether you buy the powder, solution, inner bark, or whole food.

Zinc. This mineral is fairly effective to help heal gut permeability and wounds. It is often used to bolster the immune system. Food sources include chicken, red meat, and certain cereals. Dose: Take 8 to 11 mg per day.

SPECIAL FOODS/SUPPLEMENTS FOR THE IMMUNE SYSTEM

Supplements that support the immune system can help to prevent us from falling into the "immune ditch." Astragalus (herb), vitamin C, and ginger are helpful. Long-chain omega-3 fish oils contain fatty acids that work as antioxidants and help to boost the immune system.[2] They work directly on specific white cells called B cells.

Various herbs and spices have been around for thousands of years in Southeast Asia.

Turmeric. This spice is used for its immune-boosting powers, antiseptic effect, and anti-inflammatory properties. The active ingredient is curcumin (see the next entry).

Curcumin. This extract from turmeric comes in many forms. It can be used as an anti-inflammatory and antioxidant. It is effective for joint inflammation. It is difficult to absorb, so buy a high-quality product such as Meriva that is more bioavailable to the body and does not irritate the gut.

Garlic. Garlic contains chemicals that can kill harmful bacteria and suppress their growth without causing antibiotic resistance. Garlic is not a substitute for antibiotics when treating serious infections such as blood infections or pneumonia. Garlic is best used as a support and means of preventing infections.

Ginger. This root is thought to break down accumulated toxins in the body. It may boost the immune system by preventing illness and infection, and it also has anti-inflammatory effects. Some cultures consider it a thermoregulator as it promotes sweating, which can aid with symptoms of colds and flus.

Omega-3 oils. Whether plant- or fish-based, these oils are a great antioxidant and stabilize the mast cell membranes of our immune system. When these cells burst, they release histamine which is responsible for inflammation (itchy eyes, runny nose). Omega-3 oil is also good for brain and heart health.

Seaweed. Kelp, nori, and other types of seaweed contain iodine and are helpful for thyroid function. If you are taking thyroid medications, do not supplement with more iodine.

Fermented foods. Kombucha, kefir, sauerkraut, yogurt, vinegars, and pickles provide natural sources of beneficial bacteria (probiotics) to help balance our microbiome. Almost every culture has some fermented foods in their diet.

CoQ10 (ubiquinone). This natural antioxidant is made in the body and is also found in food. It is called the "sparkplug" for our body motor. Our heart muscle uses coQ10 in large supplies. Many drugs, such as statin drugs, deplete coQ10.

Notes

PREFACE

1   Beckman T. Citations for "60–90% of all doctor's office visits are
     for stress-related ailments and complaints." LinkedIn. 2016 Apr 5.
     Available from: https://www.linkedin.com/pulse/citations-90-all-
     doctors-office-visits-stress-related-tom-beckman. Accessed 2019
     Jun 13.

1. MIND YOUR MIND

1   Phineas Gage is the first recorded case of a brain injury causing a
     change in personality and, at the time, he was studied by neurol-
     ogists and psychologists. His case is often referenced in medical
     and psychological texts. For more of his story, read Macmillan
     M. Phineas Gage—Unravelling the myth. Psychologist. 2008 Sep;
     21:828–831.
2   Nasrallah HA. Brain and mind assessment in psychiatry. Current
     Psychiatry. 2013 Mar; 12(3):8–9.
3   Journal Psyche Blog. Freud's model of the human mind. No date.
     Available from: http://journalpsyche.org/understanding-the-
     human-mind. Accessed 2020 Feb 24.
4   Lipton BH. The biology of belief: unleashing the power of conscious-
     ness, matter & miracles. Carlsbad, CA: Hay House; 2016.

5 Crum A. Change your mindset, change the game. TEDxTraverseCity. [Video] 2014 Oct 15. Available from: https://www.youtube.com/watch?v=0tqq66zwa7g. Accessed 2020 Feb 3.

6 A large research study called Adverse Childhood Experiences (ACE) was conducted by Kaiser Permanente and the Centers for Disease Control and Prevention (CDC) and found that childhood trauma was associated with health and social problems and even early death. More information and major findings are on the CDC website: https://www.cdc.gov/violenceprevention/acestudy/about.html. Accessed 2020 Feb 3.

7 Dweck CS. Mindset: the new psychology of success. London: Robinson; 2012.

8 Clay RA. Don't cry over spilled milk—the research on why it's important to give yourself a break. CE Corner. 2016 Sep; 47(8):70. Available from: https://www.apa.org/monitor/2016/09/ce-corner. Accessed 2020 Feb 3.

9 Psychology Today. What is mindfulness? No date. Available from: http://www.psychologytoday.com/us/basics/mindfulness. Accessed 2020 Feb 3.

2. MIND YOUR BRAIN

1 Bailey R. An introduction to hormones. ThoughtCo. 2018 Nov 4. Available from: https://www.thoughtco.com/hormones-373559. Accessed 2019 Jun 16.

2 National Institutes of Health. Why is the BRAIN initiative needed? No date. Available from: https://braininitiative.nih.gov/about/overview. Accessed 2019 Nov 26.

3 Estroff Marano H. Our brain's negative bias. Psychology Today. 2003 Jun 20. Available from: https://www.psychologytoday.com/us/articles/200306/our-brains-negative-bias. Accessed 2020 Feb 3.

4 Hanson R. Hardwiring happiness: the new brain science of contentment, calm, and confidence. New York: Harmony; 2013.

5 Mel Robbins. 10 ways to change your mindset right now. 2018 Dec. Available from: https://www.dropbox.com/s/ukkislm0rf32ojk/ 10WaysToChangeYourMindset.pdf. Accessed 2019 Jun 17.

6 Bergland, C. The neuroscience of savoring positive emotions. Psychology Today. 2015 Jul 24. Available from: https://www. psychologytoday.com/us/blog/the-athletes-way/201507/the-neuroscience-savoring-positive-emotions. Accessed 2019 Nov 26.

7 Dr. Norman Doidge details many fascinating examples of neuroplasticity in: Doidge N. The brain that changes itself: stories of personal triumph from the frontiers of brain science. New York: Penguin Books; 2007.

8 Castillo M. Boosting your brain, part 1: the couch potato. Am J Neuroradiol. 2013 Apr; 34(4):693-695. doi: 10.3174/ajnr.A3189.

3. MIND YOUR BREATH

1 Li P, Janczewski WA, et al. The peptidergic control circuit for sighing. Nature. 2016 Feb 8; 530:293-297. doi: 10.1038/nature16964.

2 Benson H, Klipper MZ. The relaxation response. New York: William Morrow; 2000.

3 Kabat-Zinn J. Wherever you go, there you are: mindfulness meditation in everyday life. New York: Hachette Books; 2005.

4 Yackle K, Schwarz LA, et al. Breathing control center neurons that promote arousal in mice. Science. 2017 Mar 31; 355(6332):1411-1415. Available from: doi: 10.1126/science.aai7984.

5 Bhasin MK, Dusek JA, et al. Relaxation response induces temporal transcriptome changes in energy metabolism, insulin secretion and inflammatory pathways. PLOS ONE. 2013 May 1; 8(5):e62817. doi: 10.1371/journal.pone.0062817.

6 GenomeAlberta. Gene expression in meditative and yogic practices. Genomics Blog. 2015 Nov 6. Available from: http://genomealberta. ca/genomics/gene-expression-in-meditative-and-yogic-practices. aspx. Accessed 2020 Feb 24.

4. MIND YOUR GUT

1   Gershon MD. The second brain: a groundbreaking new under-
    standing of nervous disorders of the stomach and intestine. New
    York: Harper Perennial; 1999. See also Hadhazy, A. Think twice:
    how the gut's "second brain" influences health and well-being.
    Scientific American. 2010 Feb 12. Available from: https://www.
    scientificamerican.com/article/gut-second-brain/. Accessed
    2020 Feb 3.

2   Clapp M, Aurora N, et al. Gut microbiota's effect on mental health:
    the gut-brain axis. Clin Pract. 2017 Sep 15; 7(4):987. doi: 10.4081/
    cp.2017.987.

3   Peirce JM, Alviña K. The role of inflammation and the gut micro-
    biome in depression and anxiety. J Neurosci Res. 2019 May 29;
    97(10):1223-1241. doi: 10.1002/jnr.24476.

4   Pincock S. Nobel Prize winners Robin Warren and Barry Mar-
    shall. Lancet. 2005 Oct 22; 366(9465):1429. doi: 10.1016/
    S0140-6736(05)67587-3.

5   Centers for Disease Control and Prevention. *Helicobacter pylori*: fact
    sheet for health care providers. 1998 Jul. Available from: https://
    stacks.cdc.gov/view/cdc/40603. Accessed 2020 Feb 3.

6   Levenstein S, Rosenstock S, et al. Psychological stress increases risk
    for peptic ulcer, regardless of *Helicobacter pylori* infection or use of
    nonsteroidal anti-inflammatory drugs. Clin Gastroenterol Hepatol.
    2015 Mar; 13(3):498-506.

7   Qin H-Y, Cheng C-W, et al. Impact of psychological stress on irritable
    bowel syndrome. World J Gastroenterol. 2014 Oct 21; 20(39):14126-
    14131. doi: 10.3748/wjg.v20.i39.14126.

8   Park SH, Videlock EJ, et al. Adverse childhood experiences are asso-
    ciated with irritable bowel syndrome and gastrointestinal symptom
    severity. Neurogastroenterol Motility. 2016 Aug; 28(8):1252-1260.
    doi: 10.1111/nmo.12826.

9   Oligschlaeger Y, Yadati T, et al. Inflammatory bowel disease: a
    stressed "gut/feeling." Cells. 2019 Jun; 8(7):659. doi: 10.3390/
    cells8070659.

10   Kumamoto CA. Inflammation and gastrointestinal Candida
colonization. Curr Opin Microbiol. 2011 Aug; 14(4): 386–391.
doi: 10.1016/j.mib.2011.07.015.

11   A treatment protocol used by doctors who practice functional medicine as outlined by the Institute for Functional Medicine (https://
www.ifm.org/). Functional medicine concerns itself with the how
and why of illness in order to restore health rather than control
symptoms.

12   Ivan Pavlov is the father of classical conditioning. In one of his most
famous experiments, he rang a bell each time he fed a dog. Eventually, the dog salivated when the bell rang, whether Pavlov fed the dog
or not.

13   Chong PP, Chin V K, et al. The microbiome and irritable bowel
syndrome—a review on the pathophysiology, current research and
future therapy. Front Microbiol. 2019 Jun 10; 10:1136. doi: 10.3389/
fmicb.2019.01136.

14   Underwood E. Your gut is directly connected to your brain, by
a newly discovered neuron circuit. ScienceMag. 2018 Sep 20.
Available from: https://www.sciencemag.org/news/2018/09/
your-gut-directly-connected-your-brain-newly-discovered-
neuron-circuit. Accessed 2020 Feb 3.

5. MIND YOUR MOVEMENT

1   ScienceDaily. Leg exercise is critical to brain and nervous system
health. 2018 May 23. Available from: https://www.sciencedaily.
com/releases/2018/05/180523080214.htm. Accessed 2020 Feb 3.

2   Ratey J, Hagerman E. Spark: the revolutionary new science of exercise and the brain. New York: Little, Brown & Company; 2008,
56. See also: LaMothe K. Exercise, movement, and the brain.
Psychology Today. 2015 Nov 30. Available from: https://www.
psychologytoday.com/us/blog/what-body-knows/201511/exercise-
movement-and-the-brain. Accessed 2020 Feb 3.

3   Stults-Kolehmainen M A, Sinha R. The effects of stress on physical activity and exercise. Sports Med. 2014 Jan; 44(1):81–121. doi:

10.1007/s40279-013-0090-5. See also: Leguizamon B. Can your stress hurt your fitness progress? InBody. 2018 Nov 21. Available from: https://inbodyusa.com/blogs/inbodyblog/can-your-stress-hurt-your-fitness-progress/. Accessed 2020 Feb 3.

4   Bennabi D, Vandel P, et al. Psychomotor retardation in depression: a systematic review of diagnostic, pathophysiologic, and therapeutic implications. BioMed Res Internat. 2013; Article ID 158746. doi: 10.1155/2013/158746.

5   J Nat Cancer Inst. Sedentary behavior increases the risk of certain cancers. 2014 Jul; 106(7):dju206. doi: 10.1093/jnci/dju206.

6   Meira LB, Bugni JM, et al. DNA damage induced by chronic inflammation contributes to colon carcinogenesis in mice. J Clin Invest. 2008 Jun; 118(7):2516–2525. doi: 10.1172/JCI35073.

7   Plotnikoff RC, Costigan SA, et al. Factors associated with higher sitting time in general, chronic disease, and psychologically-distressed, adult populations: findings from the 45 & Up Study. PLOS ONE. 2015 Jun 3; 10(6):e0127689. doi: 10.1371/journal.pone.0127689.

8   Pew Research Center. The future of well-being in a tech-saturated world. 2018 Apr 17. Available at: http://www.elon.edu/docs/e-web/imagining/surveys/2018_survey/Elon_Pew_Digital_Life_and_Well_Being_Report_2018_Expanded_Version.pdf. Accessed 2020 Feb 3.

9   Harvard Health Publishing. Obesity: unhealthy and unmanly. Harvard Men's Health Watch. 2011 Mar. Available from: https://www.health.harvard.edu/mens-health/obesity-unhealthy-and-unmanly. Accessed 2020 Feb 3.

10 PennState News. Kinesiology class connects motivation and exercise through research. 2010 May 26. Available from: https://news.psu.edu/story/167008/2010/05/26/kinesiology-class-connects-motivation-and-exercise-through-research. Accessed 2020 Feb 3.

11 Armstrong B. How exercise affects your brain. Scientific American. 2018 Dec 26. Available from: https://www.scientificamerican.com/article/how-exercise-affects-your-brain/. See also: Armstrong B. How exercise affects your brain. Quick and Dirty Tips. 2018 Oct 30. Available from: https://www.quickanddirtytips.com/health-fitness/exercise/how-exercise-affects-your-brain. Accessed 2020 Feb 3.

12 U.S. Department of Health and Human Services. Physical activity guidelines for Americans. Last reviewed 2019 Feb 1. Available from: https://www.hhs.gov/fitness/be-active/physical-activity-guidelines-for-americans/index.html. Accessed 2020 Feb 3.

13 Moderate aerobic activity includes brisk walking, swimming, dancing, etc. If you are engaging in moderate aerobic activity, you should be able to talk but not have enough breath to sing.

14 Vigorous aerobic activity includes running, jumping rope, playing soccer, etc. If you are engaging in vigorous aerobic activity, you are not able to carry on a conversation with someone else, as you will not have enough breath.

15 Harvard School of Public Health. Physical activity guidelines: how much exercise do you need? 2013 Nov 20. Available from: https://www.hsph.harvard.edu/nutritionsource/2013/11/20/physical-activity-guidelines-how-much-exercise-do-you-need/. Accessed 2020 Feb 3.

16 Mel Robbins. The five elements of the 5 second rule. 2018 Apr 25. Available from: https://melrobbins.com/blog/five-elements-5-second-rule. Accessed 2020 Feb 24.

17 Qi L, Kobayashi M, et al. Effects of forest bathing on cardiovascular and metabolic parameters in middle-aged males. Evid Based Complement Alternat Med. 2016; 2016:2587381. doi: 10.1155/2016/2587381.

18 Harvard sociologist Amy Cuddy's research on power posing has been controversial. See: Perry S. Is "power posing" back? MinnPost. 2018 Mar 30. Available from: https://www.minnpost.com/second-opinion/2018/03/power-posing-back/. Accessed 2020 Feb 3. I believe power poses have a positive effect on some people's emotional state. What do you have to lose by trying it?

19 Harvard Health Publishing. Exercising to relax. Harvard Men's Health Watch. 2018 Jul 13. Available from: https://www.health.harvard.edu/staying-healthy/exercising-to-relax. Accessed 2020 Feb 3.

20 Kohl HW III, Cook HD, eds. Physical activity, fitness, and physical
    education: effects on academic performance. Chapter 4 in: Educat-
    ing the student body: taking physical activity and physical education
    to school. Washington, DC: Committee on Physical Activity and
    Physical Education in the School Environment; Food and Nutri-
    tion Board; Institute of Medicine; National Academies Press; 2013.
    Available from: https://www.ncbi.nlm.nih.gov/books/NBK201501/.
    Accessed 2020 Feb 3.

21 Heijnen S, Hommel B, et al. Neuromodulation of aerobic exer-
    cise: a review. Front Psychol. 2016 Jan 7; 6:1890. doi: 10.3389/
    fpsyg.2015.01890.

22 Pignolo RJ. Exceptional human longevity. Mayo Clinic
    Proceedings. 2019 Jan; 94(1):110-124. Available from: https://www.
    mayoclinicproceedings.org/article/S0025-6196(18)30792-4/
    fulltext. Accessed 2020 Feb 3.

6. MIND YOUR HEART

1   Atrial natriuretic peptide (ANP), made in the atria, and brain natri-
    uretic peptide (BNP), made in the ventricles, are naturally secreted
    by the heart. They help regulate fluid and blood pressure in the heart.

2   Saver JL. Time is brain—quantified. Stroke. 2006 Jan; 37:263-266.
    Available from: https://www.ahajournals.org/doi/pdf/10.1161/01.
    STR.0000196957.55928.ab. Accessed 2020 Feb 3.

3   McCurry J. Japanese woman "dies from overwork" after logging 159
    hours of overtime in a month. Guardian. 2017 Oct 5. Available from:
    https://www.theguardian.com/world/2017/oct/05/japanese-
    woman-dies-overwork-159-hours-overtime. Accessed 2020 Feb 3.

4   Whitworth JA, Williamson PM, et al. Cardiovascular consequences
    of cortisol excess. Vasc Health Risk Manag. 2005 Dec; 1(4): 291-299.
    doi: 10.2147/vhrm.2005.1.4.291.

5   Friedman MD, Rosenman RH. Association of specific overt behav-
    ior pattern with blood and cardiovascular findings. JAMA. 1959;
    169(12):1286-1296. doi: 10.1001/jama.1959.03000290012005.

6   This result likely holds true for women too, but we still need more research to confirm it.

7   Ford DE, Mead LA, et al. Depression is a risk factor for coronary artery disease in men: the precursors study. Arch Intern Med. 1998; 158(13):1422–1426. doi: 10.1001/archinte.158.13.1422.

8   Centers for Disease Control and Prevention. High blood pressure. Last reviewed 2020 Jan 28. Available from: https://www.cdc.gov/bloodpressure/faqs.htm. Accessed 2020 Mar 29.

9   Kloner RA, Leor J, et al. Population-based analysis of the effect of the Northridge Earthquake on cardiac death in Los Angeles County, California. J Am College Cardiol. 1997 Nov; 30(5):1174–1180. doi: 10.1016/S0735-1097(97)00281-7.

10 Saver JL. Time is brain—quantified. Stroke. 2006 Jan; 37:263–266. Available from: https://www.ahajournals.org/doi/pdf/10.1161/01.STR.0000196957.55928.ab. Accessed 2020 Feb 3.

11 Centers for Disease Control and Prevention. Stroke. Last reviewed 2020 Feb 19. Available from: https://www.cdc.gov/stroke/index.htm. Accessed 2020 Mar 29.

12 Komamura K, Fukui M, et al. Takotsubo cardiomyopathy: pathophysiology, diagnosis and treatment. World J Cardiol. 2014 Jul 26; 6(7):602–609. doi: 10.4330/wjc.v6.i7.602.

13 Blumenthal JA, Sherwood A, et al. Enhancing cardiac rehabilitation with stress management training: a randomized, clinical efficacy trial. Circulation. 2016 Mar 21; 133(14):1341–1350. doi: 10.1161/CIRCULATIONAHA.115.018926.

14 Orth-Gomér K, Schneiderman N, et al. Stress reduction prolongs life in women with coronary disease: the Stockholm Women's Intervention Trial for Coronary Heart Disease (SWITCHD). Circ Cardiovasc Qual Outcomes. 2009 Jan; 2(1):25–32. doi: 10.1161/CIRCOUTCOMES.108.812859.

15 McCraty R. Science of the heart, volume 2: exploring the role of the heart in human performance, an overview of research conducted by the HeartMath Institute. 2016 Feb. doi: 10.13140/RG.2.1.3873.5128.

16 Nichols H. What are the leading causes of death in the US?
    Medical News Today. 2019 Jul 4. Available from: https://www.
    medicalnewstoday.com/articles/282929.php. Accessed 2019 Sep 4.

7. MIND YOUR SLEEP

1   Eugene A R, Masiuk J. The neuroprotective aspects of sleep.
    MEDtube Sci. 2015 Mar; 3(1):35–40.

2   Eugene Aserinsky was at the forefront of sleep research as a PhD
    candidate at the University of Chicago. He is considered one of the
    founders of modern sleep research, and we continue to use his meth-
    ods with the EEG to study sleep.

3   National Sleep Foundation. What happens when you sleep? No date.
    Available from: https://www.sleepfoundation.org/articles/what-
    happens-when-you-sleep. Accessed 2020 Feb 24.

4   Schwartz T. Sleep is more important than food. Harvard Business
    Review. 2011 Mar 3. Available from: https://hbr.org/2011/03/sleep-
    is-more-important-than-f. Accessed 2020 Feb 3.

5   National Sleep Foundation. National Sleep Foundation recommends
    new sleep times. 2015 Feb 2. Press release. Available from: https://
    www.sleepfoundation.org/press-release/national-sleep-foundation-
    recommends-new-sleep-times. Accessed 2020 Feb 3.

6   American Sleep Apnea Association. Sleep health terminology: the
    difference between insomnia and sleep deprivation. 2017 Jun 9.
    Available from: https://www.sleepapnea.org/sleep-health-
    terminology-insomnia-versus-sleep-deprivation/. Accessed 2020
    Feb 3.

7   Centers for Disease Control and Prevention. 1 in 3 adults don't
    get enough sleep. Available from: https://www.cdc.gov/media/
    releases/2016/p0215-enough-sleep.html. Accessed 2020 Feb 3. See
    also: Vriend J, Corkum P. Clinical management of behavioral insom-
    nia of childhood. Psychol Res Behav Manag. 2011; 4:69–79. doi:
    10.2147/PRBM.S14057.

8   Weeks, BS. MIT study: cell phone radiation linked to insomnia, con-
     fusion, headaches, depression. 2008 Jan 20. Available from: http://
     weeksmd.com/2008/01/mit-study-cell-phones-and-insomnia/.
     Accessed 2020 Feb 3.

9   Harvard Health Publishing. Sleep and mental health. Harvard Men-
     tal Health Letter. Available from: https://www.health.harvard.edu/
     newsletter_article/sleep-and-mental-health. Accessed 2020 Feb 3.

10   National Sleep Foundation. Aging and sleep. 2009 Dec. Available
     from: https://www.sleepfoundation.org/articles/aging-and-sleep.
     Accessed 2020 Feb 3.

11   National Institute of Neurological Disorders and Stroke. Restless
     legs syndrome fact sheet. 2019 Aug 13. Available from: https://www.
     ninds.nih.gov/Disorders/Patient-Caregiver-Education/Fact-Sheets/
     Restless-Legs-Syndrome-Fact-Sheet. Accessed 2019 Nov 28.

12   ScienceDaily. Sleep loss dramatically lowers testosterone in healthy
     young men. 2011 Jun 1. Available from: https://www.sciencedaily.
     com/releases/2011/05/110531162142.htm. Accessed 2020 Feb 3.

13   Wolf E, Kuhn M, et al. Synaptic plasticity model of therapeutic sleep
     deprivation in major depression. Sleep Med Rev. 2016 Dec; 30:53–62.
     doi: 10.1016/j.smrv.2015.11.003.

14   Consumer Reports. Why Americans can't sleep: people are
     desperate for shut-eye, and turning to drugs, supplements and high-
     tech gadgets for help. 2016 Jan 14. Available from: https://www.
     consumerreports.org/sleep/why-americans-cant-sleep/. Accessed
     2019 Sep 11.

15   Breus MJ. How can binaural beats help you sleep better? Psychology
     Today. 2018 Oct 11. Available from: https://www.psychologytoday.
     com/us/blog/sleep-newzzz/201810/how-can-binaural-beats-help-
     you-sleep-better. Accessed 2020 Feb 3.

16   Wolfson E. The rise of Ambien: why more Americans are taking
     the sleeping pill and why the numbers matter. HuffPost. 2013 Jul 8.
     Available from https://www.huffpost.com/entry/ambien_
     b_3223347. Accessed 2020 Feb 3.

8. MIND YOUR IMMUNE SYSTEM

1   D'Acquisto F. Affective immunology: where emotions and the immune response converge. Dialogues Clin Neurosci. 2017 Mar; 19(1):9–19. Available from: https://www.ncbi.nlm.nih.gov/pmc/articles/PMC5442367/. Accessed 2020 Feb 3.

2   Mattes E, McCarthy S, et al. Maternal mood scores in mid-pregnancy are related to aspects of neonatal immune function. Brain Behav Immun. 2009 Mar; 23(3):380–388. doi: 10.1016/j.bbi.2008.12.004.

3   Strachan DP. Hay fever, hygiene, and household size. British Med J. 1989; 299:1259–1260. doi: 10.1136/bmj.299.6710.1259.

4   Zheng P, Zeng B, et al. Gut microbiome remodeling induces depressive-like behaviors through a pathway mediated by the host's metabolism. Molecular Psychiatry. 2016; 21:786–796. Available from https://www.nature.com/articles/mp201644. Accessed 2020 Feb 3.

5   Health Knowledge. Measures of disease frequency and disease burden. No date. Available from: https://www.healthknowledge.org.uk/e-learning/epidemiology/practitioners/measures-disease-frequency-burden. Accessed 2020 Feb 3.

6   Fairweather D, Rose NR. Women and autoimmune diseases. Emerg Infectious Dis. 2004 Nov; 10(11):2005–2011. doi: 10.3201/eid1011.040367.

7   Manzel A, Muller DN, et al. Role of "Western" diet in inflammatory autoimmune diseases. Curr Allergy Asthma Rep. 2014 Jan; 14(1):404. doi: 10.1007/s11882-013-0404-6.

8   Daruna JH. Introduction to psychoneuroimmunology. 2nd ed. London: Elsevier, Inc.; 2012.

9   Besedovsky L, Lange T, Born J. Sleep and immune function. Pflugers Arch – Eur J Physiol. 2012 Jan; 463(1): 121–137, doi: 10.1007/s00424-011-1044-0.

10 Chopra D, Tanzi R. The healing self: a revolutionary new plan to supercharge your immunity and stay well for life. New York: Harmony Books; 2018.

11 Epel ES, Puterman E, et al. Meditation and vacation effects have an impact on disease-associated molecular phenotypes. Transl Psychiatry. 2016 Aug 30; 6(8):e880. doi: 10.1038/tp.2016.164.

12 Black DS, Slavich GM. Mindfulness meditation and the immune system: a systematic review of randomized controlled trials. Ann NY Acad Sci. 2016 Jun; 1373(1):13–24. doi: 10.1111/nyas.12998.

13 Mount Sinai Health System. Systems biology research study reveals benefits of vacation, meditation. ScienceDaily. 2016 Aug 30. Available from: https://www.sciencedaily.com/releases/2016/08/160830091815.htm. Accessed 2020 Feb 25.

14 Stenström CH, Minor MA. Evidence for the benefit of aerobic and strengthening exercise in rheumatoid arthritis. Arthritis Care & Res. 2003 Jun 15; 49(3):428–434, doi: 10.1002/art.11051.

15 Clarke CD. How gratitude actually changes your brain and is good for business. Thrive Global. 2018 Feb 7. Available from: https://thriveglobal.com/stories/how-gratitude-actually-changes-your-brain-and-is-good-for-business/. Accessed 2020 Feb 3.

16 Achor S. Positive intelligence. Harvard Business Review. 2012 Jan–Feb. Available from: https://hbr.org/2012/01/positive-intelligence. Accessed 2020 Apr 5. See also: Lyubomirsky S, King L, Diener, E. The benefits of frequent positive affect: does happiness lead to success? Psychol Bull. 2005 Oct 31; 131(6): 803–855. doi: 10.1037/0033-2909.131.6.803 .

APPENDIX B: SUPPLEMENTS

1 Scheer R, Moss D. Dirt poor: have fruits and vegetables become less nutritious? Scientific American. 2011 Apr 27. Available from: https://www.scientificamerican.com/article/soil-depletion-and-nutrition-loss/. Accessed 2020 Feb 3.

2 Gurzell EA, Teague H, et al. DHA-enriched fish oil targets B cell lipid microdomains and enhances ex vivo and in vivo B cell function. J Leukocyte Biol. 2013 Apr; 93(4):463–470. doi: 10.1189/jlb.0812394.

Selected Bibliography

BOOKS

Amen DG. Change your brain, change your life. New York: CMI/ Premier Education Solutions; 2011.

Bredesen DE, LeMonnier J. The end of Alzheimer's: the first program to prevent and reverse cognitive decline. Waterville, ME: Thorndike Press; 2018.

Brown B. The gifts of imperfection: let go of who you think you're supposed to be and embrace who you are. Charleston, SC: Instaread Summaries; 2014.

Chopra DM. Perfect health. Milsons Point, NSW: Random House Australia; 2001.

Chopra DM. Quantum healing: exploring the frontiers of mind/body medicine. New York: Bantam Books; 2015.

Crowley C, Lodge HS. Younger next year for women: live strong, fit, and sexy—until you're 80 and beyond. New York: Workman Publishing; 2007.

Cuddy AJC. Presence: bringing your boldest self to your biggest challenges. New York: Little Brown and Company; 2015.

Dienstfrey H. Where the mind meets the body. New York: Harper Collins; 1991.

Dispenza J. You are the placebo: making your mind matter. Carlsbad, CA: Hay House, Inc.; 2015.

Dispenza J, Amen DG. Breaking the habit of being yourself. Carlsbad, CA: Hay House; 2015.

Doidge N. The brain's way of healing: remarkable discoveries and recoveries from the frontiers of neuroplasticity. Brunswick, Victoria, Australia: Scribe Publications; 2017.

Domar AD, Dreher H. Healing mind, healthy woman. London: Thorsons; 1997.

Fritz MA, Speroff L. Clinical gynecologic endocrinology and infertility. Philadelphia: Lippincott Williams & Wilkins; 2010.

Gaby A. Nutritional medicine. Concord, NH: Fritz Perlberg Publishing; 2017.

Hanson R, Hanson F. Resilient: find your inner strength. London: Rider Books; 2018.

Hanson R, Mendius R. Buddha's brain: the practical neuroscience of happiness, love, and wisdom. Oakland, CA: New Harbinger Publications; 2009.

Junger A. Clean gut: the breakthrough plan for eliminating the root cause of disease and revolutionizing your health. New York: HarperCollins; 2015.

Maté G. When the body says no. Toronto: Vintage Canada; 2012.

McGraw PC. Self matters: creating your life from the inside out. New York: Free Press; 2001.

Myers A. The autoimmune solution: prevent and reverse the full spectrum of inflammatory symptoms and diseases. New York: HarperOne; 2017.

Northrup C. The wisdom of menopause: creating physical and emotional health during the change. New York: Bantam Books; 2012.

Perlmutter D, Loberg K. Brain maker: the power of gut microbes to heal and protect your brain—for life. London: Yellow Kite; 2015.

Pert CB. Molecules of emotion: why you feel the way you feel. New York: Scribner; 2003.

Rankin L. Mind over medicine. Carlsbad, CA: Hay House; 2013.

Robbins M. The 5 second rule: transform your life, work, and confidence with everyday courage. USA: Savio Republic; 2017.

Siegel DJ. The mindful brain: reflection and attunement in the cultivation of well-being. New York: W.W. Norton; 2007.

Talbott SM. The cortisol connection: why stress makes you fat and ruins your health—and what you can do about it. Alameda, CA: Hunter House; 2007.

Winter WC. The sleep solution: why your sleep is broken and how to fix it. New York: Berkley; 2017.

MAGAZINE ARTICLES

Brewer J. The science of bad habits. Mindful magazine. 2018 Apr; 60–63. Available for purchase from: https://www.mindful.org/issue/april-2018/.

Finkel M. While we sleep, our mind goes on an amazing journey. National Geographic. 2018 Aug; 40–77. Available from: https://www.nationalgeographic.com/magazine/2018/08/science-of-sleep/. Accessed 2020 Feb 24.

Maté G. Inside the ayahuasca experience: when shamanism meets psychotherapy. 2018 Sep/Oct. Psychotherapy Networker. Available from: https://psychotherapynetworker.org/magazine/article/2311/inside-the-ayahuasca-experience/. Accessed 2020 Feb 24.

Ricard M, Lutz A, Davidson RJ. Mind of the meditator. Scientific American: MIND. Special ed. 2018 Mar; 27(1s): 90–97. Available for purchase from: https://www.scientificamerican.com/magazine/special-editions/2018/special-editions-volume-27-issue-1s/.

Smookler E. Focus on the good. Mindful magazine. 2018 Apr; 30–32. Available for purchase from: https://www.mindful.org/issue/april-2018/.

SCIENTIFIC ARTICLES

Bartlett DB, Willis LH, et al. Ten weeks of high-intensity interval walk training is associated with reduced disease activity and improved innate immune function in older adults with rheumatoid arthritis:

a pilot study. Arthritis Res Ther. 2018; 20(1):127. doi: 10.1186/s13075-018-1624-x.

Blumenthal J, Fredrikson M, et al. Aerobic exercise reduces levels of cardiovascular and sympathoadrenal responses to mental stress in subjects without prior evidence of myocardial ischemia. Am J Cardiol. 1990 Jan; 65(1):93–98. doi: 10.1016/0002-9149(90)90032-v.

Bonnet MH, Arand DL. Hyperarousal and insomnia: state of the science. Sleep Med Rev. 2010 Feb; 14(1):9–15.

Bunt J, Boileau R, et al. Sex and training differences in human growth hormone levels during prolonged exercise. J Appl Physiol. 1986 Nov; 61(5):1796–1801. doi: 10.1152/jappl.1986.61.5.1796.

Buono M, Yeager J, Hodgdon J. Plasma adrenocorticotropin and cortisol responses to brief high-intensity exercise in humans. J Appl Physiol. 1986 Oct; 61(4):1337–1339. doi: 10.1152/jappl.1986.61.4.1337.

Chen E, Miller GE. Stress and inflammation in exacerbations of asthma. Brain Behav Immun. 2007 Nov; 21(8):993–999. doi: 10.1016/j.bbi.2007.03.009.

Cheungsamarn S, Rattanamongkolgul S, et al. Reduction of atherogenic risk in patients with type 2 diabetes by curcuminoid extract: a randomized controlled trial. J Nutr Biochem. 2014 Feb; 25(2):144–150. doi: 10.1016/j.jnutbio.2013.09.013.

Christian LM. Stress and immune function during pregnancy: an emerging focus in mind-body medicine. Curr Dir Psychol Sci. 2015 Feb; 24(1):3–9. doi: 10.1177/0963721414550704.

Cianci R, Pagliari D, et al. The microbiota and immune system crosstalk in health and disease. Mediators Inflamm. 2018; 2018:2912539. doi: 10.1155/2018/2912539.

Corcoran P. Use it or lose it—the hazards of bed rest and inactivity. West J Med. 1991 May; 154:536–538. Available from: https://www.ncbi.nlm.nih.gov/pmc/articles/PMC1002823/pdf/westjmed00105-0054.pdf. Accessed 2020 Feb 25.

Craft LL. Exercise and clinical depression: examining two psychological mechanisms. Psychol Sport Exercise. 2005 Mar; 6(2):151–171. doi: 10.1016/j.psychsport.2003.11.003.

Dimsdale J E. Psychological stress and cardiovascular disease. J
  Am Coll Cardiol. 2008 Apr 1; 51(13):1237–1246. doi: 10.1016/j.
  jacc.2007.12.024.

Ding S, Jiang H, Fang J. Regulation of immune function by polyphenols.
  J Immunol Res. 2018; 2018:1264074. doi: 10.1155/2018/1264074.

Dishman R, Berthoud H, et al. Neurobiology of exercise. Obesity. 2012
  Sep 6; 14(3):345–356. doi: 10.1038/oby.2006.46.

Du M, Chen Z J. DNA-induced liquid phase condensation of cGAS
  activates innate immune signaling. Science. 2018 Aug 17;
  361(6403):704–709. doi: 10.1126/science.aat1022.

Elliott D E, Siddique S S, Weinstock J V. Innate immunity in disease. Clin
  Gastroenterol Hepatol. 2014 May; 12(5):749–755. doi: 10.1016/j.
  cgh.2014.03.007.

Ersche K D, Lim T-V, et al. Creature of habit: a self-report measure of
  habitual routines and automatic tendencies in everyday life. Pers
  Individ Dif. 2017 Oct 1; 116:73–85. doi: 10.1016/j.paid.2017.04.024.

Francino M P. Antibiotics and the human gut microbiome: dysbioses and
  accumulation of resistances. Front Microbiol. 2016 Jan 12; 6:1543.
  doi: 10.3389/fmicb.2015.01543.

Guimarães M R, Leite F R, et al. Curcumin abrogates LPS-induced
  proinflammatory cytokines in RAW 264.7 macrophages. Evidence for novel mechanisms involving SOCS-1, -3 and p38 MAPK.
  Arch Oral Biol. 2013 Aug 22; 58(10):1309–1317. doi: 10.1016/j.
  archoralbio.2013.07.005.

Hato T, Dagher P C. How the innate immune system senses trouble and
  causes trouble. Clin J Am Soc Nephrol. 2015 Aug; 10(8):1459–1469.
  doi: 10.2215/CJN.04680514.

Hirtosu C, Tufik S, Andersen M L. Interactions between sleep, stress,
  and metabolism: from physiological to pathological conditions.
  Sleep Sci. 2015 Nov; 8(3):143–152. doi: 10.1016/j.slsci.2015.09.002.

Jacks D, Sowash J, et al. Effect of exercise at three intensities on salivary
  cortisol. Med Sci Sports Exercise. 1999 May; 31(Suppl.):S266. doi:
  10.1097/00005768-199905001-01290.

Kamada N, Rogler G. The innate immune system: a trigger for many chronic inflammatory intestinal diseases. Inflamm Intest Dis. 2016 Jul; 1(2):70–77. doi: 10.1159/000445261.

Kenny MJ, Ganta CK. Autonomic nervous system and immune system interactions. Compr Physiol. 2014 Jul; 4(3):1177–1200. doi: 10.1002/cphy.c130051.

Kindermann W, Schnabel A, et al. Catecholamines, growth hormone, cortisol, insulin, and sex hormones in anaerobic and aerobic exercise. Eur J Appl Physiol. 1982; 49(3):389–399. doi: 10.1007/bf00441300.

Labzin LI, Heneka MT, Latz E. Innate immunity and neurodegeneration. Annu Rev Med. 2018 Jan; 69:437–449. doi:10.1146/annurev-med-050715-104343.

Li J, Perez-Perez GI. *Helicobacter pylori* the latent human pathogen or an ancestral commensal organism. Front Microbiol. 2018 Apr 3; 9:article 609. doi: 10.3389/fmicb.2018.00609.

Mayer EA. The neurobiology of stress and gastrointestinal disease. Gut. 2000 Dec 1; 47(6):861–869. doi: 10.1136/gut.47.6.861.

Mollazadeh H, Cicero AFG, et al. Immune modulation by curcumin: the role of interleukin-10. Crit Rev Food Sci Nutr. 2017 Sep 6; 59(1):89–101. doi: 10.1080/10408398.2017.1358139.

Moss D, Shaffer F. The application of heart rate variability biofeedback to medical and mental health disorders. Biofeedback. 2017; 45(1):2–8.

Nabkasorn C, Miyai N, et al. Effects of physical exercise on depression, neuroendocrine stress hormones and physiological fitness in adolescent females with depressive symptoms. Eur J Pub Health. 2006 Apr; 16(2):179–184. doi: 10.1093/eurpub/cki159.

Navegantes KC, de Souza Gomes R, et al. Immune modulation of some autoimmune diseases: the critical role of macrophages and neutrophils in the innate and adaptive immunity. J Transl Med. 2017; 15(1):36. doi: 10.1186/s12967-017-1141-8.

Neu J, Rushing J. Cesarean versus vaginal delivery: long-term infant outcomes and the hygiene hypothesis. Clin Perinatol. 2011 Jun; 38(2):321–331. doi: 10.1016/j.clp.2011.03.008.

Power G, Dalton B, et al. Motor unit number estimates in masters
  runners : use it or lose it? Med Sci Sports Exercise. 2010 Sep;
  42(9):1644–1650. doi: 10.1249/mss.0b013e3181d6f9e9.

Pruett SB. Stress and the immune system. Pathophysiology. 2003 May;
  9(3):133–153. doi: 10.1016/s0928-4680(03)00003-8.

Puertollano MA, Puertollano E, et al. Dietary antioxidants: immunity
  and host defense. Curr Top Med Chem. 2011; 11(14):1752–1766.

Puterman E, Lin J, et al. The power of exercise: buffering the effect of
  chronic stress on telomere length. PLOS ONE 2010 May; 5(5):e10837.
  doi: 10.1371/journal.pone.0010837.

Radosevich P, Nash J, et al. Effects of low- and high-intensity exercise
  on plasma and cerebrospinal fluid levels of ir-β-endorphin, ACTH,
  cortisol, norepinephrine and glucose in the conscious dog. Brain
  Research. 1989 Sep 25; 498(1):89–98. doi: 10.1016/0006-8993(89)
  90402-2.

Russo MA, Santarelli DM, O'Rourke D. The physiological effects of slow
  breathing in a healthy human. Breathe (Sheff). 2017 Dec; 13(4):298–
  309. doi: 10.1183/20734735.009817.

Scully D, Kremer J, et al. Physical exercise and psychological well
  being: a critical review. Brit J Sports Med. 1998; 32(2):111–120. doi:
  10.1136/bjsm.32.2.111.

Shaykhiev R, Crystal RG. Innate immunity and chronic obstructive pulmonary disease: a mini-review. Gerontol. 2013; 59(6):481–489. doi:
  10.1159/000354173.

Simpson RJ, Kunz H, et al. Exercise and the regulation of immune functions. Prog Mol Biol Transl Sci. 2015; 135:355–380. doi: 10.1016/
  bs.pmbts.2015.08.001.

Smith SM, Vale WW. The role of the hypothalamic-pituitary-adrenal
  axis in neuroendocrine responses to stress. Dialogues Clin Neurosci. 2006 Dec; 8(4):383–395. Available from: https://www.ncbi.nlm.
  nih.gov/pmc/articles/PMC3181830/.

Starkie R, Ostrowski S, et al. Exercise and IL-6 infusion inhibit
  endotoxin-induced TNF-α production in humans. FASEB Journal.
  2003 May; 17(8):884–886. doi: 10.1096/fj.02-0670fje.

Tettamanti L, Caraffa AI, et al. Different signals induce mast cell inflammatory activity: inhibitory effect of vitamin E. J Biol Regul Homeost Agents. 2018; 32(1):13–19.

Traustadóttir T, Bosch P, Matt K. The HPA axis response to stress in women: effects of aging and fitness. Psychoneuroendocrinol. 2005; 30(4):392–402. doi:10.1016/j.psyneuen.2004.11.002.

Wadley AJ, Holliday A, et al. Preliminary evidence of reductive stress in human cytotoxic T cells following exercise. J Appl Physiol. 2018 Aug; 125(2):586–595. doi:10.1152/japplphysiol.01137.2017.

Yan W. Impact of prenatal stress and adulthood stress on immune system: a review. Biomed Res. 2012; 23(3):315–320. Available from: https://www.alliedacademies.org/articles/impact-of-prenatal-stress-and-adulthood-stress-on-immune-system-a-review.pdf.

ONLINE ARTICLES AND VIDEOS

American Heart Association. Stress and heart health. Last reviewed 2014 Jun 17. Available from: https://www.heart.org/en/healthy-living/healthy-lifestyle/stress-management/stress-and-heart-health. Accessed 2020 Feb 24.

American Psychological Association. Stress weakens the immune system. 2006 Feb 23. Available from: https://www.apa.org/research/action/immune. Accessed 2020 Feb 24.

Bailey R. An introduction to hormones. ThoughtCo. 2019 Sep 1. Available from: https://www.thoughtco.com/hormones-373559. Accessed 2020 Feb 24.

Burschka J. What your breath could reveal about your health. TED@ Merck KGAA, Darmstadt, Germany. [Video] 2018 Nov. Available from: https://www.ted.com/talks/julian_burschka_what_your_breath_could_reveal_about_your_health. Accessed 2020 Feb 24.

Centers for Disease Control and Prevention. Adverse childhood experiences. Last reviewed 2019 Apr 2. Available from: https://www.cdc.gov/violenceprevention/acestudy/index.html. Accessed 2020 Feb 24.

Centers for Disease Control and Prevention. High blood pressure, frequently asked questions. Last reviewed 2020 Jan 28. Available from: https://www.cdc.gov/bloodpressure/faqs.htm. Accessed 2020 Feb 24.

Fehrs L. Muscle memory, trauma and massage therapy. Institute for Integrative Healthcare. 2013 Aug 1. Available from: https://www.integrativehealthcare.org/mt/muscle-memory-trauma-and-massage-therapy. Accessed 2020 Feb 24.

Gray N. Omega-3 backed to boost immune response, not just battle inflammation: study. Nutra Ingredients. 2013 Apr 1. Available from: https://www.nutraingredients.com/Article/2013/04/02/Omega-3-backed-to-boost-immune-health-not-just-battle-inflammation. Accessed 2020 Feb 24.

Harvard Health Publishing. Men and depression. Harvard Mental Health Letter. 2006 Nov. Available from: https://www.health.harvard.edu/newsletter_article/Men_and_depression. Accessed 2020 Feb 24.

Harvard Health Publishing. Stress and your heart. Harvard Women's Health Watch. 2013 Dec. Available from: https://www.health.harvard.edu/heart-health/stress-and-your-heart. Accessed 2020 Feb 24.

Heart Matters. Feeling stressed? Research shows how stress can lead to heart attacks and stroke. No date. Available from: https://www.bhf.org.uk/informationsupport/heart-matters-magazine/news/behind-the-headlines/stress-and-heart-disease. Accessed 2020 Feb 24.

How Sleep Works. Available from: https://www.howsleepworks.com. Accessed 2020 Feb 24.

Howes L. Heal your body with your mind: Dr. Joe Dispenza. [Video] 2018 Aug 12. Available from: https://www.youtube.com/watch?reload=9&v=Mggxik0ZN80. Accessed 2020 Feb 24.

Howes L. Your thoughts will heal or kill you with Marisa Peer and Lewis Howes. [Video] 2018 Sep 18. Available from: https://www.youtube.com/watch?v=V4TqTkks7AA. Accessed 2020 Feb 24.

Hudson T. Cortisol and sleep: the HPA axis activity connection. Integrative Therapeutics. 2017 Feb 6. Available from: https://www.integrativepro.com/Resources/Integrative-Blog/2017/Cortisol-and-Sleep. Accessed 2020 Feb 24.

James M. React vs. respond. What's the difference? Psychology Today blog. 2016 Sep 1. Available from: https://www.psychologytoday.com/ca/blog/focus-forgiveness/201609/react-vs-respond. Accessed 2020 Feb 24.

Lane E. What is muscle memory? Get back in the gym and gains will return fast—thanks to muscle memory. Men's Health. 2015 Jun 24. Available from: http://www.menshealth.co.uk/building-muscle/what-is-muscle-memory. Accessed 2020 Feb 24.

Manitoba Trauma Information & Education Centre. Post-traumatic growth. No date. Available from: http://trauma-recovery.ca/resiliency/post-traumatic-growth/. Accessed 2020 Feb 24.

McGonigal K. How to make stress your friend. TEDGlobal 2013. [Video] 2013 Jun. Available from: https://www.ted.com/talks/kelly_mcgonigal_how_to_make_stress_your_friend. Accessed 2020 Feb 24.

Newman J. How breast milk protects newborns. KellyMom. Updated 2018 Jan 2. Available from: https://kellymom.com/pregnancy/bf-prep/how_breastmilk_protects_newborns/. Accessed 2020 Feb 24.

Rifkin R. How shallow breathing affects your whole body. Headspace.com. No date. Available from: https://www.headspace.com/blog/2017/08/15/shallow-breathing-whole-body/. Accessed 2020 Feb 24.

Robbins T. Why we do what we do. TED2006. [Video] 2006 Feb. Available from: https://www.ted.com/talks/tony_robbins_asks_why_we_do_what_we_do. Accessed 2020 Feb 24.

Roberts C. Natural ways to boost your immune system. Active Beat. Updated 2020 Jan 20. Available from: https://www.activebeat.com/diet-nutrition/10-natural-ways-to-boost-your-immune-system/10/. Accessed 2020 Feb 24.

Sadhguru. The four parts of the mind—Vinita Bali with Sadhguru. [Video] 2015 May 27. Available from: https://www.youtube.com/watch?v=PHVHMiPiKao. Accessed 2020 Feb 24.

ScienceDaily. How we form habits, change existing ones. Society for Personality and Social Psychology. 2014 Aug 8. Available from: https://www.sciencedaily.com/releases/2014/08/140808111931.htm. Accessed 2020 Feb 24.

The Well Project. Understanding the immune system. 2020 Jan 15. Available from: https://www.thewellproject.org/hiv-information/understanding-immune-system. Accessed 2020 Feb 24.

WebMD. Stress and asthma. No date. Available from: http://www.webmd.com/asthma/guide/stress-asthma#1. Accessed 2020 Feb 24.

Wolkin J. Train your brain to boost your immune system. 2016 Mar 23. Available from: https://www.mindful.org/train-brain-boost-immune-system/. Accessed 2020 Feb 24.

Index

Figures indicated by page numbers in italics

Abdul (hypertension case study), 174–75

absorption, of nutrients, 92, 94

acid reflux, 101, 111. *See also* gastroesophageal reflux disease; heartburn

acne, 90

active immunity, 223–25

adaptability, 207–8

adaptogenic herbs, 278–79

adenoids, 227, 230

adiponectin, 137

adrenal glands, 46–48, *47*, 168, 203

adrenaline: activation by sympathetic nervous system, 42–43, *45*, *47*, 73; breathing and, 72; chronic stress and, 52; exercise and, 156, 256; heart health and, 168, 172, 179–80; immune system and, 232; inflammatory bowel disease and, 104–5; pain and, 133; panic attacks and, 77; sleep disorders and, 197; stroke and, 179

adrenocorticotropic hormone (ACTH), 46

aerobic (cardio) exercise, 124, 125–26, 128, 144, 256, 290nn13–14

alcohol, 95, 111, 112, 185, 189, 202, 212

aldosterone, 47

allergies: allergic asthma, 74; to food, 220, 240–41; immune system and, 224

alveoli, *67*, 68, 71

Am I Hungry? (app), 118

Alzheimer's disease, 16, 123, 157. *See also* dementia

amygdala, 46, 53, 138

anaerobic (strength training) exercise, 124, 144, 256

anemia, 203, 220

anger, 7, 72, 170, 176, 179

antibiotics and antibiotic-resistant diseases, 103, 111, 233–34

antibodies, 222–23, 224–25, 226, 245

anus, *93*, 94

anxiety, 24, 65, 103–4, 183, 198, 278–79

apnea. *See* obstructive sleep apnea

Aristotle, 160

arrhythmia, 179–80

arteries, 164, 173

arthritis, rheumatoid, 90, 235, 236, 237–39, 247

Aserinsky, Eugene, 194, 293n2

aspirin, 111

assessments: for gut health, 110, 112, 268–72; in REFRAME toolkit, 259–60. *See also* examinations, health

asthma, 73–76

atrial natriuretic peptide (ANP), 291n1

attitude. *See* mindset

autoimmune (AI) diseases, 234–37, 236, 241–42. *See also* immune system

autonomic ganglion, 40, 41

autonomic nervous system (ANS): breath and, 69–70; chronic stress and, 44, 49–50; cognitive reframing and, 252; controlled breathing for re-setting, 80–82, 84; guided breathing exercises for, 85; gut and, 100; heart and, 161, 179; immune system and, 222, 232; involuntary movement and, 40, 126; overview, 39, 39, 40–42, 41, 47. *See also* anxiety; parasympathetic nervous system; sympathetic nervous system

bacteria: dysbiosis, 102–3, 234; *Helicobacter pylori*, 102, 111;

microbiome (intestinal flora), 96–98, 99; repopulation of, 113–14, 243, 257, 274, 280–81

basal ganglia, 126, 127

B cells, 230, 231, 235, 281

beliefs, 21, 28, 34, 35. *See also* mindset

Benson, Herbert, 78–79, 81, 82, 86–87, 253

beta-carotene, 276

betaine hydrochloride, 279–80

bile, 94

binaural beats, 211

biofeedback, 182–83, 213

bloating, 89, 103, 240

blood disorders, 220

blood pressure, high (hypertension), 173–75

blood vessels, 164–65

body integration, 129–30

body memory, 16

bone marrow, 222, 224, 226, 227, 230

bradycardia, 179

brain, 36–63; introduction and conclusion, 36–39, 62–63; adrenal glands, 46–48, 47, 168, 203; aerobic exercise and, 125–26; amygdala, 46, 53, 138; autonomic nervous system, 39, 40–42, 41; benefits of a healthy brain, 61–62; breathing and, 69–72, 70; central and peripheral nervous systems, 39, 39, 41; cultivation of, 54–61; electrical brain waves, 54; gut and, 90–91, 98–99,

100; heart and, 165–69, *167*;
hippocampus, 46, 53, 138,
155; homeostasis, 42–43;
hypothalamic-pituitary-
adrenal (HPA) axis, 46, 47, 203,
279; hypothalamus, 45–46, 47,
155, 190, *192*, 193; immune
system and, 222; left-brain vs.
right-brain, 61; limbic system,
46, 115, 138; mapping brain
function, 11; mind and, 3,
9–11, 17, 18–19; movement
and, 126–27, 128–29, 145;
musculoskeletal system and,
125; neurobic exercises, 59–
60; parasympathetic nervous
system, 43–44; pituitary gland,
45–46, 47, 193; prefrontal
cortex, 10, 50, 129, 148; self-
assessment, 36–37; sleep and,
194; slowing down nervous system, 60–61; somatic nervous
system, *39*, 40; story, savor,
smile technique, 56–57; stress
and, 5, 38–39, 47, 49–54; suprachiasmatic nucleus, 190–92,
192, 193; sympathetic nervous
system, 42–43; taking in the
good, 55; training the brain,
57–59
brain-derived neurotrophic factor
(BDNF), 61, 154–55
brain fog, 89
brain natriuretic peptide (BNP),
291n1
brainstem, *41*, 50, 69, 70, 86, *125*,
166, *167*

breast milk, 223, 224
breath, 64–88; introduction and
conclusion, 64–66, 88; anatomy of respiratory system, 66,
67; asthma, 73–75; author's
story, 78–80, 82; automatic vs.
conscious breathing, 69–72,
70; benefits of controlled
breathing, 85–87; breath, mind,
word (BMW) meditation, 82–84,
117, 199, 253–55, 263–64; case
studies, 75–76, 78; controlled
breathing, 84–85, 255; cultivation of, 80–85; emotions
and, 72, 79; guided breathing
exercises, 85; hyperventilation
syndrome and panic attacks,
76–77; metabolic control of
breathing, 70–71; normal
breathing, 68–69; reactions vs.
responses, 73; re-setting autonomic nervous system, 80–82,
84; self-assessment, 64–65;
shallow breathing, 64, 72; sighing, 71; stress and, 72–80
breath, mind, word (BMW) meditation, 82–84, 117, 199, 253–55,
263–64
Breathe (app), 85
bronchi, *67*, 68
bronchitis, 219
Buddhify (app), 211

caffeine, 111, 112, 185, 189, 212
Calm (app), 85
cancer, 22, 101, 103, 111, 123, 137,
186, 236

capillaries, *162*, 164

carbon dioxide, 68, 70-71, 76-77, 164

cardiac nerves, *167*

cardio (aerobic) exercise, 124, 125–26, 128, 144, 256, 290nn13-14

cardiovascular system, *162*. *See also* heart

Carol (mindset case study), 22–25

cells: cell-signaling theory, 130–31; memory within, 16

central fat obesity, 134. *See also* weight gain and obesity

central nervous system (CNS), 39, *39, 41*

cerebellum, *125*, 126, 127

cerebrospinal fluid, 194

Chopra, Deepak, 28

chronic obstructive pulmonary disease (COPD), 203

chronic pain, 27, 99, 133, 139, 155, 198, 199

chyme, 93–94

circadian rhythm, 54, 156, 190–92, *191, 192*, 198

cognitive behavioral therapy (CBT), 58–59, 212-13

cognitive reframing, 251–52. *See also* REFRAME toolkit

colds, 76, 89, 105, 157, 234, 243, 282

colitis, ulcerative, 104, 235, *236*

colostrum, 223

Comey, Rob, 212, 214

compassion, self-, 30-31

compressed sleep, 213-14

concentration, 207-8

conscious mind, 12-13

consciousness, 12, 16

constipation, 89, 103, 108, 140, 235

controlled breathing, 84-85, 85-87, 255. *See also* breath

controlled stimulus therapy (CST), 213

coQ10 (ubiquinone), 283

coronary arteries, 164-65, 176

corticotropin-releasing factor (CRF), 46

cortisol: activation by sympathetic nervous system, 43, 46, 47, 73; body arousal and, 193, 207; brain and, 52-53; damage from too much, 48; emotional eating and, 116; exercise and, 153-54, 156, 256; functions of, 47; heart health and, 168, 172; immune system and, 224, 232; inflammatory bowel disease and, 104-5; insulin resistance and, 137; muscle and, 134; pain and, 133; panic attacks and, 77; peptic ulcers and, 102; psychomotor retardation and, 135; sleep disorders and, 54, 197, 198; stroke and, 179; weight gain and, 206

cortisol manager (supplement), 279

covert stress, 48

cramping, 220, 240

C-reactive protein, 243, 246

criticism, self-, 7

Crohn's disease, 104, 235, *236*, 275, 277

curcumin, 282
curiosity, 31
Cushing's syndrome, 169-70
cytokines, 222, 229, 244-45

Daruna, Jorge H., 242
Debbie (immune system case study), 237-39
decision-making, 147-49
dehydroepiandrosterone (DHEA), 43, 193
Dekker, Thomas, 188
dementia, 54, 99, 157, 190. *See also* Alzheimer's disease
depression, 99, 104, 135, 141, 156, 171-72, 181-82
diabetes: chronic stress and, 2; Cushing's syndrome and, 169; diet and, 184; exercise and, 157, 185; fatigue and, 203; heart damage from, 176; Relaxation Response and, 86; sedentary lifestyle and, 137; sleep and, 54, 198, 207; Type 1 diabetes, 236; visceral body fat and, 134
diaphragm, 67, 68-69, 70, 72, 79, 82
diarrhea, 89, 103-4, 105-6, 110, 220, 240
diet: anti-inflammatory diet, 111, 243; 5R gut program, 110-14, 258; heart-healthy diet, 184-85; recommended, 273-74; in REFRAME toolkit, 257-58; stress and, 53. *See also* eating; food allergies; supplements

digestion, 92-93, 109, 114, 119, 220
digestive enzymes, 94, 98, 112, 114, 280
dopamine, 52, 135, 202, 247
dreams, 196
Dweck, Carol: *Mindset*, 19-20
dysbiosis, 102-3, 234

ear infections, 219
eating: emotional eating, 115-16; mindful eating, 116-18; reflexive eating, 37; in REFRAME toolkit, 257-58. *See also* diet; food allergies
eczema, 90, 220
electrical brain waves, 54
emotional eating, 115-16
emotional freedom technique (EFT), 58-59
emotions: breath and, 72, 79; emotional health, 7-8; neuroimaging, 15; vs. thoughts, 34, 170. *See also* mind
endorphins, 44, 83, 87, 155, 156, 199, 245
enterochromaffin cells, 109
enterocytes, 94-95, 95
epiglottis, 66, 67
epinephrine, 203
esophagus, 92-93, 93, 101
estrogen, 204
examinations, health, 262-63. *See also* assessments
exercise. *See* movement

fat, visceral, 134, 137-38. *See also* weight gain and obesity fatigue, 27, 90, 122, 202–3, 204, 220

fermented foods, 113, 243, 257, 274, 282–83

fight-or-flight response. *See* sympathetic nervous system

5R gut program, 110–14, 258

five-second rule, 148–49

fixed mindset, 19–20. *See also* mindset

flexibility (stretching) exercise, 125, 144, 256

flu, 76, 89, 157, 234, 243, 282

focus, 147

food allergies, 220, 240–41

food sensitivities (intolerances), 90, 220, 240

forest bathing, 152

forgiveness, self-, 30–31

Freud, Sigmund, 14

Friedman, Meyer, 170

functional medicine, 242, 288n11. *See also* integrative medicine

Gage, Phineas, 10–11, 284n1

gallbladder, 93, 94

gamma-aminobutyric acid (GABA), 73, 87, 154, 215, 278

garlic, 282

gas, 89, 118

gastric juices, 44, 93, 103

gastroesophageal reflux disease (GERD), 101, 116. *See also* heartburn

gastrointestinal (GI) tract, 93. *See also* gut

ghrelin, 137, 206

ginger, 282

goals, SMART, 146

gratitude, 247–48

Graves' disease (hyperthyroidism), 235, 236

growth hormone, 193, 195, 245

growth mindset, 19–20. *See also* mindset

gut, 89–120; introduction and conclusion, 89–91, 119–20; anatomy and evolution of, 91–92, 93; author's story, 107–9; as barrier to disease, 94–98, 95; benefits of healthy gut, 109, 118–19; brain and, 90–91, 98–99, 100; case study, 105–7; cultivation of, 109–18; digestion and absorption process, 92–94; dysbiosis, 102–3, 234; emotional eating, 115–16; exercise and, 118; 5R gut program, 110–14, 258; gastroesophageal reflux disease (GERD), 101, 116; gut health assessment, 110, 112, 268–72; immune system and, 96, 221, 232–33, 241; inflammation, 100–101; inflammatory bowel disease (IBD), 104–5, 107; irritable bowel syndrome (IBS), 103–4; leaky gut syndrome, 95–96; microbiome (intestinal flora), 96–98, 99; mindful eating, 116–18; peptic ulcers, 102; self-assessment, 89–90; serotonin in, 53, 107, 109, 119, 257; stress and, 53,

100–109, 111; supplements for, 113, 114, 279–81

gut-associated lymphatic tissue (GALT), 95, 96, 97, 98, 227, 228, 244

Hanson, Rick, 55

Hashimoto's disease (hypothyroidism), 235, 236

hay fever, 220, 225

headaches, 89

Headspace (app), 85, 211

health mindset: author's story, 27–28, 34; benefits of, 33–34; characteristics of, 20–21, 25–27; cultivation of, 25–32; curiosity and openness, 31; mindfulness, 31–32; passion, 30; persistence, 30; positive role models, 29–30; self-assessment, 28; self-compassion and kindness, 30–31; SODA technique, 28–29, 261. See also mindset

heart, 159–87; introduction and conclusion, 159–61, 186–87; anatomy of, 161–63, 162; arrhythmia, 179–80; author's story, 180; benefits of healthy heart, 186; case studies, 174–75, 177–78; as communication network, 165–70; cultivation of, 181–86; depression and, 171–72, 181–82; diet for, 184–85; electrical pathways, 165; exercise and, 185; heart attack, 165, 168, 176–78; hypertension (high blood pressure), 173–75; neurological pathways, 165–69, 167;

personality types and, 170–71; regulating heart rate, 182–83; self-assessment, 159–60; sleep and, 185–86; smoking and, 183–84; stress and, 166, 168, 169–70, 170–81; stroke, 178–79; takotsubo cardiomyopathy, 181; as transportation network, 164–65

heart attack, 165, 168, 176–78

heartburn, 89, 101, 111, 280. See also gastroesophageal reflux disease

heart disease, 54, 123, 134, 171–72, 181–82, 183–84, 185, 203

HeartMath Institute, 183

Helicobacter pylori, 102, 111

herbs, adaptogenic, 278–79

high blood pressure (hypertension), 173–75

hippocampus, 46, 53, 138, 155

Hippocrates, 89, 119, 219

HIV. See human immunodeficiency virus

homeostasis, 42–44, 118, 193, 227

hormone fluctuations, 203–4. See also specific hormones

human immunodeficiency virus (HIV), 246–47

human leukocyte antigen (HLA), 96

hygiene: hygiene hypothesis, 225; sleep hygiene, 211–12

hypersomnia, 204

hypertension (high blood pressure), 173–75

hyperthyroidism (Graves' disease), 235, 236

hyperventilation syndrome (HVS), 65, 76–78

hypervigilance, 138–39, 235

hypnosis, sleep, 210

hypothalamic-pituitary-adrenal (HPA) axis, 46, 47, 203, 279

hypothalamus, 45–46, 47, 155, 190, *192*, 193

hypothyroidism (Hashimoto's disease), 235, *236*

ibuprofen, 111

illness mindset, 21–22. *See also* mindset

immune system, 219–50; introduction and conclusion, 219–21, 249–50; active immunity, 223–25; anatomy of, 226–28, 227; antibiotic-resistant diseases, 233–34; author's story, 243–44; autoimmune (AI) diseases, 234–37, *236*, 241–42; barriers, 228; benefits of, 248; brain and, 222; case study, 237–39; cultivation of, 241–48; definition, 221–22; diet for, 243; dysbiosis, 102–3, 234; environment and, 242–43; exercise and, 247; as "floating brain," 232; food allergies, 240–41; general responders, 229; gratitude and positivity and, 247–48; gut and, 96, 221, 232–33, 241; hygiene hypothesis, 225; immune tolerance, 222; innate immunity, 228–29; meditation and, 245–47; origins of, 222–26; passive immunity, 223; psychoneuroimmunology, 222,

242; self-assessment, 219–20; sleep and, 208, 244–45; specific responders, 229–31; stress and, 224, 232–41, *233*; supplements for, 281–83; as three-tiered defense system, 226–31; vaccinations, 226

immune tolerance, 222

inactivity (sedentary lifestyle), 53–54, 122–23, 131, 137, 138, 141, 149–51. *See also* movement

inflammation: anti-inflammatory diet, 111, 243; autoimmune diseases and, 234–35; effects of, 53, 98–99, 101; exercise and, 156–57; immune system and, 229; overview, 100–101

inflammatory bowel disease (IBD), 89, 104–5, 107

injuries, from movement, 136

innate immunity, 228–29

Insight Timer (app), 211

insomnia, 200–201, 209, 212–13, 274. *See also* sleep

insulin and insulin resistance, 137–38, 206–7, 234

integrative medicine, 2, 3, 186, 241, 249, 263. *See also* functional medicine

intelligence, 15

intestinal flora. *See* microbiome

intestines, *93*, 94

intolerances, food, 240

involuntary movement, 40, 126

iron, 97, 202, 257, 274

irritable bowel syndrome (IBS), 89, 103–4

James, William, 7
Jane (mindset case study), 22–25
Jason (heart attack case study), 177–78
jellyfish, 92
Joe (gut case study), 105–7
joint stiffness, 122, 134–35, 220
Judy (movement case study), 149–51

Kabat-Zinn, Jon, 81, 253
karoshi (overwork death), 169
Katz, Lawrence: *Keep Your Brain Alive*, 59–60
Keller, Helen, 159
kindness, 30–31
kinesiology, 123
Kuttner, Leora, 210

large intestine, *93, 94*, 104
leaky gut syndrome, 95–96
leptin, 137, 206
leverage, 147
L-glutamine, 280
limbic system, 46, 115, 138
Lipton, Bruce, 16
liver, *93, 94*, 97, 118, 156, 207, 276
L-theanine, 279
lungs, *67, 68, 162*
lupus, 235, 236, *236*
lymphatic system, 226, 230. *See also* gut-associated lymphatic tissue (GALT)
lymph nodes, 227

magnesium, 274, 277, 278
Marshall, Barry, 102

medical system, 2–4. *See also* functional medicine; integrative medicine
medications, sleep, 215–16
meditation: apps for, 85, 211; breath, mind, word (BMW) meditation, 82–84, 117, 199, 253–55, 263–64; breathing and, 80; focus and, 147; heart health and, 183; immune system and, 245–47; sleep and, 209–11; for training the brain, 58; walking meditation, 156. *See also* mindfulness
medulla oblongata, *41*, 69, *70*
melatonin, 83, *191*, 192–93, 198, 199, 204, 245, 278
memory: body memory, 16; in brain, 46; exercise and, 154–55; loss of, 89, 215; in muscle cells, 127–28, 132; of trauma, 138–39
mental health and illness, 7–8, 13, 99. *See also* mind
metabolic control of breathing, 70–71
metacognition, 11, 29
Michelle (asthma case study), 75–76
microbiome: development and functions, 96–98; dysbiosis, 102–3, 234; mental health and, 99; repopulation of, 113–14, 243, 257, 274, 280–81. *See also* gut
microvilli, 94
mind, 7–35; introduction and conclusion, 7–8, 14, 34–35;

in breath, mind, word (BMW) meditation, 83; conscious and unconscious minds, 12-14, 17-18; metacognition, 11, 29; mindset, 17-34; multidimensional perspective, 15-17; neuroimaging and, 15; perspectives on nature of, 11-14; relationship to brain, 3, 9-11, 17; self-assessment, 7-8. *See also* health mindset; mindset

mind-body integration: introduction, 1-6; brain, 36-63; breath, 64-88; gut, 89-120; heart, 159-87; immune system, 219-50; mind, 7-35; movement, 121-58; REFRAME toolkit, 251-64; sleep, 188-218. *See also specific topics*

Mindful Eating Tracker (app), 118

mindfulness, 31-32, 58, 116-18. *See also* meditation

mindfulness-based stress reduction (MBSR), 81-82

mindset, 17-34; author's story, 27-28, 34; case study, 22-25; definition, 17; growth vs. fixed mindset, 19-20; health mindset, 20-21, 25-34; illness mindset, 21-22; for movement, 141-43; in REFRAME toolkit, 261-62; relationship with body and brain, 18-19; self-assessment, 28; unconscious mind and, 17-18. *See also* health mindset

minerals, 277

mood, 7, 122, 141, 156, 207-8

morning routine, 36

motivation, 8, 146

motor cortex, *125*, 126, 135

motor neuron disease, 128

motor neurons, *125*, 126, 127

movement (exercise), 121-58; introduction and conclusion, 121-23, 157-58; aerobic (cardio) exercise, 124, 125-26, 128, 144, 256, 290nn13-14; anaerobic (strength training) exercise, 124, 144, 256; author's story, 139-40; benefits of, 153-57; body integration, 129-30; brain and, 126-27, 128-29, 145; breathing and, 70-71; case study, 149-51; chronic muscle pain, 138-39; communal exercise, 151; cultivation of, 141-53; exercise guidelines, 143-45; flexibility (stretching) exercise, 125, 144, 256; gut and, 118; heart health and, 185; immune system and, 247; inflammation reduction, 156-57; injuries, 136; insulin resistance and weight gain, 137-38; memory improvements, 154-55; mood and sleep, 156; muscle cell growth, 130-32; muscle memory, 127-28, 132; muscle tension and joint stiffness, 134-35; musculoskeletal system, 123-26, *125*; outdoors, 151-52; pain relief, 155; psychomotor retardation, 135-36; in REFRAME toolkit,

255–56; resilience, 130; sarcopenia (muscle wasting), 131–32,
138; sedentary lifestyles, 141;
seeking help with, 152; self-
assessment, 121–22; for slowing
down nervous system, 60–61;
SMUFLD formula, 145–49, 256;
staying positive, 152–53; stress
and, 53–54, 132–41, 153–54;
voluntary and involuntary
movement, 126
mucous membranes, 226, 228
multidimensional mind, 15–17
multiple sclerosis, 128, 235, 236,
236
muscles: brain and, 127, 128; cell
growth, 130–32; chronic muscle
pain, 138–39; cortisol and, 134;
exercise, 124; memory within,
127–28, 132; sarcopenia (muscle
wasting), 131–32, 138; tension
within, 134–35
musculoskeletal system, 123–26,
125. See also movement
Muse (headband), 85
myasthenia gravis, 236
mySleepButton (app), 211

nausea, 109, 140, 220
negative thoughts, 7, 8, 48–49, 58,
261. See also brain; mindset
nerves, 39
neural crest, 90
neurobic exercises, 59–60
neurocardiology, 168
neurogastroenterology, 98–99
neuroimaging, 15

neuro-linguistic programming
(NLP), 58–59
neurologists, 11–12
neurons, 40, 41, 51, 51–52, 53, 61,
86, 109, 129, 196, 207. See also
motor neurons
neuroplasticity, 52–53, 57–58
Nhất Hạnh, Thích, 64
no, saying, 61
"nocebo" effect, 22
norepinephrine, 52, 154, 203
nutritional deficiencies, 90

obesity. See weight gain and
obesity
obstructive sleep apnea (OSA), 188,
201–2
omega-3 oils, 282
openness, 31
overt stress, 48
oxytocin, 73, 193

pain, 27, 99, 133, 139, 155, 198, 199
pancreas, 93, 94, 118, 206–7
panic attacks, 64, 76–78
paradoxical intention therapy,
214–15
parasympathetic nervous system
(PNS; rest-and-digest response):
activation, 80, 87, 246; eating
and, 257; gut and, 100, 109,
118; heart and, 168; homeostasis, 42–44; immune system and,
221, 246; neuroplasticity and,
58; overview, 39, 40, 41, 43–44,
45, 47; re-setting, 209, 253
passion, 30
passion flower, 278

passive immunity, 223
Pavlov, Ivan, 115, 288n12
peptic ulcers, 102, 116
perfectionism, 8
perimenopause, 204
peripheral nervous system, 39, 39
peristalsis, 93, 98, 109, 119
persistence, 30
personality, 10–11, 170–71
phantom pain, 139
phosphatidylserine, 278, 279
phrenic nerve, 68–69, 70
pineal gland, 192, 192
pituitary gland, 45–46, 47, 193
platelet counts, low, 179, 220
pleura, 67, 68
pneumonia, 219, 282
pons, 41, 69, 70
positive thinking, 25, 33, 247–48.
    See also mindset
post-traumatic stress disorder
    (PTSD), 53, 139. See also trauma
practical knowledge, 15–16
prebiotics, 97, 113, 274, 280
prefrontal cortex, 10, 50, 129, 148
premenstrual syndrome (PMS),
    204
probiotics, 97, 113–14, 243, 280–81
progesterone, 204, 205–6
prolactin, 193
psoriasis, 220, 235, 236
psychiatrists, 13
psychologists, 12–13
psychomotor retardation, 135–36
psychoneuroimmunology, 222,
    242
pulmonary circulation, 162, 163

Ramón y Cajal, Santiago, 36
Ratey, John, 129
reactions, vs. responses, 73
REFRAME toolkit, 251–64;
    introduction, 251–53; assess,
    259–60; examine, 262–63;
    exercise, 255–56; food, 257–58;
    how to use, 263–64; mindset,
    261–62; re-set, 253–55; rest,
    258–59
rejection, feelings of, 8
relaxation and rest: in 5R gut pro-
    gram, 114; for immune system,
    245–47; in REFRAME toolkit,
    258–59; for sleep, 209–11. See
    also sleep
Relaxation Response, 81, 82,
    86–87, 253
REM (rapid eye movement) sleep,
    194, 195–96
re-set, 253–55
resilience, 130
respiratory system, 67. See also
    breath
responses, vs. reactions, 73
rest. See relaxation and rest
rest-and-digest response. See para-
    sympathetic nervous system
restless legs syndrome (RLS),
    202
rheumatoid arthritis, 90, 235, 236,
    237–39, 247
Robbins, Mel, 56, 148, 248
role models, positive, 29–30
rosacea, 90
Rosenman, Ray, 170

saliva, 92

Sam (hyperventilation syndrome and panic attacks case study), 78

Sarah (sleep case study), 205–6

sarcopenia (muscle wasting), 131–32, 138

seaweed, 282

sedentary lifestyle (inactivity), 53–54, 122–23, 131, 137, 138, 141, 149–51. *See also* movement

selenium, 277

self-care, difficulties with, 8

self-compassion, 30–31

self-criticism, 7

sensitivities, food, 240

serotonin: activation, 43, 73, 83–84, 87, 199, 245; effects of, 109; exercise and, 145, 154, 156; in gut, 53, 107, 109, 119, 257; from medication, 99; microbiome and, 113; stress and, 52

sex, 141

shallow breathing, 64, 72. *See also* breath

SierraSil (supplement), 277

sighing, 71

sinoatrial node, 165, *167*

sinus, 227, 228

sinus infections, 189, 219, 234

sitting, 122–23. *See also* sedentary lifestyle

skin, 226, 227, 228

skin infections, 219

sleep, 188–218; introduction and conclusion, 188–90, 217–18; author's story, 199; benefits of, 216–17; body rest and repair, 193–94; case study, 205–6; chronic pain and, 198; circadian rhythm, 54, 156, 190–92, *191*, *192*, 198; cognitive behavioral therapy (CBT), 212–13; controlled stimulus therapy (CST), 213; cultivation of, 208–16; exercise and, 156; fatigue and, 202–3; heart health and, 185–86; hormone fluctuations and, 203–4; immune system and, 208, 244–45; insomnia, 200–201, 209, 212–13, 274; medications for, 215–16; meditation for, 209–11; melatonin and other hormones, 83, 192–93, 198, 199, 204, 278; mood, concentration, and adaptability, 207–8; normal sleep cycles, 190–96; obstructive sleep apnea (OSA), 201–2; paradoxical intention therapy, 214–15; in REFRAME toolkit, 258–59; REM sleep, 194, 195–96; restless legs syndrome (RLS), 202; self-assessment, 188–89; sleep deprivation, 200; sleep hygiene, 211–12; sleep hypnosis, 210; sleep restriction therapy (SRT), 213–14; sleep-wake homeostasis, 193; for slowing down nervous system, 60; stages of, 194–96; stress and, 53, 54, 196–208; supplements for, 278; weight gain and obesity, 206–7 sleep restriction therapy (SRT), 213–14

slippery elm, 281

small intestine, 93, 94, 97

SMART goals, 146

smiling, 56–57

smoking, quitting, 183–84

SMUFLD (Smart, Motivation, Urgency, Focus, Leverage, and Decisions) formula, 145–49, 256

snore, 188, 201

SODA (Stop, Observe, Detach, Affirm) technique, 28–29, 261

somatic nervous system, 39, 39, 40

soul, 14, 16

soundwave technology, 211

spinal cord, 39, 41, 90–91, 100, 125, 126, 127, 153

spiritual scholars, 14

spleen, 226, 227, 230

stomach, 93, 93

story, savor, smile technique, 56–57, 248

strength training (anaerobic exercise), 124, 144, 256

stress: adaptive techniques, 48–49; brain effects, 5, 38–39, 47, 49–54; breath and, 72–80; definition, 44–45; gut and, 53, 100–109, 111; heart and, 166, 168, 169–70, 170–81; homeostasis, 42–44; hypothalamic-pituitary-adrenal (HPA) axis, 46, 47; immune system and, 224, 232–41, 233; movement (exercise) and, 53–54, 132–41, 153–54; overt vs. covert stress, 48; short-circuiting techniques, 54–61; significance of, 2; sleep and, 53, 54, 196–208. *See also* adrenaline; cortisol; sympathetic nervous system

stretching (flexibility exercise), 125, 144, 256

stroke, 178–79

subconscious mind, 12–13, 13–14, 17–18

supplements, 273–83; introduction, 257, 273–75; for anxiety, 278–79; fat-soluble vitamins, 276–77; for gut, 113, 114, 279–81; for immune system, 281–83; minerals, 277; for sleep, 278; water-soluble vitamins, 275

suprachiasmatic nucleus (SCN), 190–92, 192, 193

sympathetic nervous system (SNS; fight-or-flight response): activation, 38, 42–43, 72, 166; breath and, 72, 74, 79, 82; exercise and, 153–54; gut and, 98, 100, 111; heart and, 166, 168, 176; homeostasis, 42–44; immune system and, 221; irritable bowel syndrome and, 103; overview, 39, 40, 41, 47; pain and, 133; panic attacks and, 77

systemic circulation, 163, 164

tachycardia, 179

taking in the good, 55

takotsubo cardiomyopathy, 181
Tanzi, Rudolph, 247
T cells, 208, 230, 231, 247
telomeres, 246
testosterone, 203–4
thalamus, *125*, 126–27
thoughts, 34–35, 49, 170. *See also* mindset; positive thinking
thymus, 226, 227, 230
thyroid and thyroid hormone, 180, 193, 235, 282
tonsils, 227, 230
trachea, *67*, 68, 227
trauma, 12, 29, 49, 133, 138–39, 285n6. *See also* post-traumatic stress disorder
turmeric, 281

ulcerative colitis, 104, 235, *236*
ulcers, peptic, 102, 116
urgency, 146–47

vaccinations, 226
vagus nerve, *41*, 42, 69–70, *70*, 98, 109, 117, *167*, 168, 253

valerian root, 278
vasculitis, *236*
veins, 164
ventral striatum, 56
villi, 94
visceral fat, 134, 137–38. *See also* weight gain and obesity
visualization, 210–11
vitamin A, 276
vitamin B, 274, 275
vitamin C, 275, 281
vitamin D, 276
vitamin E, 276–77
voluntary movement, 40, 126

walking meditation, 156
Warren, Robin, 102
weight gain and obesity, 134, 137–38, 143, 206–7, 234
Welch, Carol, 121
Westcoast Women's Clinic for Hormone Health, 4

zinc, 277, 281